Illuminated

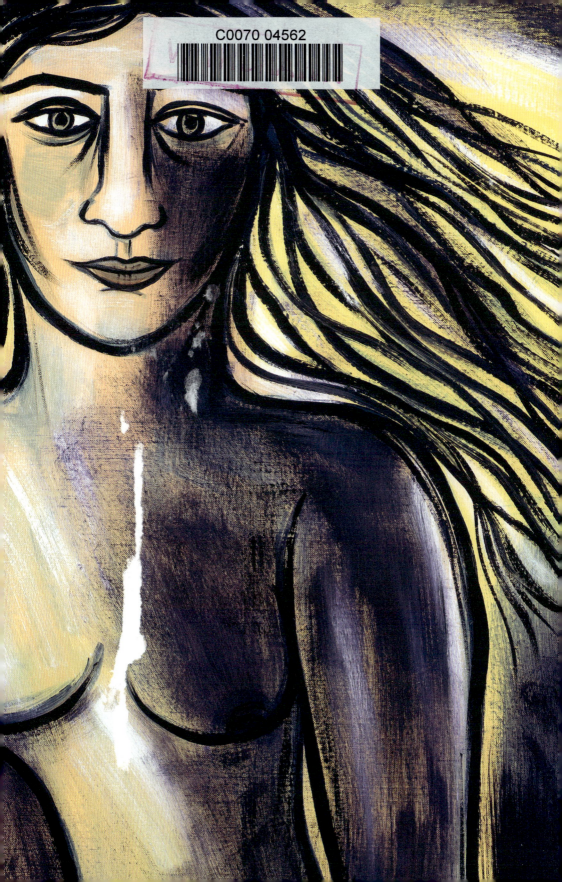

MELANIE SYKES

Autism and all the Things I've Left Unsaid

Illuminated

Harper
North

HarperNorth
Windmill Green
24 Mount Street
Manchester M2 3NX

A division of
HarperCollins*Publishers*
1 London Bridge Street
London SE1 9GF

www.harpercollins.co.uk

HarperCollins*Publishers*
Macken House, 39/40 Mayor Street Upper
Dublin 1, D01 C9W8

First published by HarperNorth in 2023

1 3 5 7 9 10 8 6 4 2

A catalogue record for this book
is available from the British Library

HB ISBN: 978-0-00-859147-2

Printed and bound in the UK using 100%
renewable electricity at CPI Group (UK) Ltd

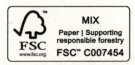

To Ligita – thank you for always being in my corner.
I love you.

'The dead stick "I", like the staff of the maypole, can be the centre of the turning world, or it can be the electric needle that picks up and relays the thronging choirs of life around it.'

Laurie Lee

Intro

I believe in destiny and I believe in timing. For years, people have asked me, 'When will you write your book?' In my late thirties I laughed it off. Too young, l thought. What have I got to share anyway, my imposter syndrome would chime? 'Not now, possibly not ever,' was my response. Then when I was in my forties it was brought up again. This time my feelings had changed; the answer was still no, but my reasoning was that I didn't want to tell the truth about my life – I was hiding too much, so frightened to tell my story in its raw form. I felt that my deepest thoughts were too dark to share, and I thought that speaking out would hurt people and possibly cause trouble for myself – perhaps ruin some of my relationships, my career and my ability to earn. I believed, if I could not tell the truth, what was the point? Why would I put out a heavily edited version of my life? Then I turned 50 and suddenly, overnight, I adopted a devil-may-care attitude, and any semblance of 'giving a fuck' seemed to desert me. Any slivers of irreverence that I'd shown historically had now almost become all of me. I came to appreciate that my life has been shared with lots of people who hold their own unique perspective, that they are entitled to, as am I to mine.

So I approached someone in the book business and after telling her some details of my life, and discussing some deep, difficult topics that I had never before shared, the response was: 'Yes, but what makes you different?', then was dismissed to think about it. Which hurt.

Not long after came my diagnosis of autism and ADHD, which lifted the lid on my life and forced me to return to the beginning. The unlocking of 'why?' that my diagnosis afforded me enabled me to drop my guard in a way that was natural but that culminated in a nervous breakdown. I was caught in a twister, and it broke every psychological bone in my body, wrung me out and ripped me apart emotionally, leaving me foetal-like on the floor, making sounds I did not recognise, coming from a place I thought I would never get back from.

Coming to terms with who I was and having an explanation for many of the decisions and behaviours over my life was freeing, but also left me stripped back and vulnerable, and it shocked me back to life, to embracing a new, more authentic existence. This book comes directly from those gaping wounds, and writing about my own personal journey has helped me immeasurably.

I woke to a question on my phone one morning from a friend: 'What is your definition of success?' My answer to this has changed over the years, and it was a good question to kick-start my day. It made me think about what 'success' means to me now. I replied: 'Success is being centred enough to know what I want, finding a comfortable way to achieve it and, most importantly, knowing that I am worthy enough to get it.'

This book has been a part of my journey back to myself, and in answer to that question posed to me a year ago, 'What makes you different?' – well, the answer is this: 'I'm different in a million ways, as we all are.' And I believe that all of those differences should be respected by everyone, but mostly by ourselves. So this book was written for me and for you. I hope you enjoy it.

Melanie x

Diagnosis

I was thrashing out ideas about the future of my magazine, *The Frank Magazine*, with a colleague when my phone pinged, intercepting the conversation. It was the clinic with the results of my autism assessment. It stopped me dead in my tracks, and I told my colleague that I just needed a minute to look at it – there was no way I could continue our conversation until I had read it.

Since autism advocate Harry Thompson had suggested I should seek a diagnosis a month or so before, I had convinced myself he was right by doing a surface mental inventory of my life. It made sense to me – the low moments, the confusing moments, my growing loneliness, my noticeable differences from others, and my pursuit of the truth were areas I had been masking. I was convinced he was right, but now, in front of me, was the truth.

I read and reread the email with a type of nervous scanning, like waiting for a job offer or exam results. It said:

'When considering all the evidence, it was agreed that Melanie's presentation meets the criteria for a diagnosis of Autism Spectrum Disorder.'

At the age of 51 I had been handed the missing piece of a complex and intricate jigsaw that was my life. I felt like I had won the lottery; it was a validation – and a huge gift. I finally could start to forgive myself for my mistakes; all my pain and baffling episodes had new meaning. I was grateful, happy and relieved – and I could not wait to tell everyone. I rang my parents, then took to social media to tell everyone else. It was a celebration.

I knew this was just the tip of the iceberg, and I knew I had work to do. Now I had to dissect my life in more detail; and to do that, I would have to go back to the beginning.

Chapter 1

I was raised in the cleft of a valley, a cotton mill town named Mossley, in Tameside, in the North West of England. (Mossley means 'a woodland clearing by a swamp or bog' – sexy, I know. Don't tell anyone …)

Mossley is nestled in the foothills of the Pennines on the edge of Saddleworth Moors, which are perhaps best known for the infamous Moors Murders in the 1960s. Green rolling hills frame steep and undulating roads, and some cobblestoned streets remain, as a reminder of bygone days. There also remain the rows of 'two-up, two-down' terraces that once housed textile workers and spinners of old. It is a place split by a thoroughfare that takes you from Yorkshire over the tops of the Pennines to our nearest major city, Manchester.

'Mossley Brew' is the town's main high street, a road that separates the 'top' from the 'bottom' of the town. These two parts feel like different entities; Bottom Mossley, where I lived for much of my childhood, was a basin through which a canal runs, dwarfed by lush green hills and the lovely stone Victorian magnificence that punctuates the landscape as you rise up to Top Mossley, where the well-to-do historically lived, and the views are suitably impressive.

The lack of horizon from the valley mentally dictated that there wasn't much outside of it. Neighbouring towns would refer to Mossley's inhabitants – us – as 'sheep shaggers', which I didn't understand as a kid and as a young adult wasn't impressed by. But with no vista or horizon to tempt you past its borders and firmly held within the hills' embrace, Mossley was the centre of my universe and, for me, there was nothing to see, conquer or acquire beyond it. I hadn't any concept of ever leaving, no desire to seek anything past it, no yearning to go too far. I still love my home town and have learned to appreciate it entirely as an adult and certainly as a mother. Being brought up there was a blessing.

While Mossley was my foundation, my mum, Wendy, came from a world away from north-west England. Mum is Anglo-Indian, born and bred in Rajasthan at a time when Anglo-Indians still bore the hallmarks of being a product of the East India Company's rule in India in the late eighteenth and early nineteenth centuries. Way back then, it was typical for British officers and soldiers to take local wives and start families, due to the lack of available English women. These Anglo-Indian children were taught the English school curriculum, given Western names, practised Christianity and were positively encouraged to see themselves as English.

Mum is the eldest of four children – her siblings being Neil, Judy and Rodney. Nana also lost a child named Gillian, who died six months after she was born. Mum remembers being told it was due to the baby developing rickets. It must have been a devastating blow to Nana, but even so, it was a loss of which I never heard her speak. Nana was beautiful, pale-skinned and delicate; Grandad, dark with thick wavy Brylcreemed hair, was tall and handsome. They were a beautiful couple. They lived in the Anglo-Indian colony in Gangapur, where Grandad worked on the railways, like his father before him — although he was unable to secure a job as a driver or mechanic due to his colour blindness, so instead he managed the workshop as a foreman for the maintenance men. They were kept very busy, not least because calls to derailment sites across north-west India were frequent due to free-roaming cows, which held revered status and sacred regard.

Nana did not work, and like many Anglo-Indian families they had Indian servants. They had a great social life in the colony; Grandad was the entertainment secretary at their local social hub, 'the institute', and would do the bingo calling on a Wednesday night and be master of ceremonies for the dances. They organised bottle and tin competitions of different descriptions where the winners would take the spoils. In addition, there were billiards tournaments and three-card gambling, and Grandpa was also a keen sportsman, loving cricket, tennis, shooting and fishing.

The only real threat to them was being robbed. Just after they were married, before they had moved to the Anglo-Indian colony, a group of intruders entered their house in the dead of night to rob them of their wedding gifts and belongings. Grandad tried to stop them, and their response was to set about him, slashing him with a dharia knife, leaving wounds on his hands, legs, face and body. Grandad's sister Sybil was a nurse, and she treated and healed his wounds, but he was left with scars on his hands where he had held them up to protect himself.

Partition of India and Pakistan perforated their relatively happy existence, and in 1947 India gained its independence, and the ripples across the country started to affect them. Suddenly the English were leaving, and the Indians were reclaiming their roles and positions in society – Indian teachers took over the schools, and all children began to learn Hindi. Like many people caught up in the decline of the British Empire, they perceived Britain to be their country, so they began to plan for the epic voyage to get here.

Paying for five of them to leave was no mean feat. The family saved and sold everything they had, and in 1961, bought five passages for just over £300 and sent over £90 ahead to Britain to help them get started on their new life. Great Britain, they believed, was their cultural heritage, and it was where they wanted to be now that their home had changed so considerably. On arrival after the seventeen-day passage to England, they contacted friends up north and found a place to live, sharing a house with many other families until they found their feet, finally settling in Mossley and getting work at the cotton mills by their home.

My dad, on the other hand, had deep roots in the north; his father, Sam Sykes, worked for the postal service, first as a postman and then as counter staff, and was a music man through and through. The Sykes family line has, for generations, been involved in the brass band community, and he was no exception – he played, conducted and composed music for brass bands.

Dad's side of the family is pretty small; his mum, Edith, had lost a baby, so Dad was an only child. I never met my paternal grandfather, as he died when Dad was about to turn nineteen. He passed at home from lung cancer and colon cancer. Dad remembers the silence in the house after his death; his father's laboured breathing had been present for some time, then suddenly it was gone. Dad was simply told his father had died and then was ushered out of the house to inform people at the post office and tell the few family members dotted around the neighbouring towns. After that, he told me, he just felt numb.

I wish I could have known Grandad. When I carried on the family tradition and played in a brass band, I played his music and I'm very proud of his achievements. Grandma suffered a stroke shortly after my Grandad died, and although she survived she only had use of one arm and her face collapsed to one side. She walked with a cane after that and used a walking frame at home.

My beautiful exotic mum and my handsome teddy boy, quiffed dad married young – when she was eighteen and he was twenty-one – which was the norm at that time. They met while working at a Timpson's shop, Mum downstairs on the repairs counter and Dad upstairs repairing the shoes. After arriving at the same time most days, they got talking, and when Dad had a week off he realised how much he had missed their chats and decided that on his return he would find out if she was single and ask her for a date. Dad finally plucked up the courage to ask, and they went to the 'pictures' to see a Western, of all things. Dad would tell me later that during this period of mild flirtation and courtship and because of his awkwardness, 'I don't know why she put up with me.'

Dad is an introverted extrovert, which I can relate to. In the right circumstances he has no problems socially; things were only difficult when he was out of his comfort zone. When he is brass banding, though, he is in his element. From the get-go, Mum was to be a brass band widow until she herself joined the band many years later.

Dad comes from a time when dyslexia was not picked up, which meant that he left school unable to read or write. When my parents were married, Mum tried to teach him, but mainly he taught himself, and after that there was no stopping him. Throughout my youth, Dad sat at the dining table with a large dictionary, writing letters to the local paper, getting involved with the community and sharing his opinions. These brilliantly, painstakingly composed letters would almost always be published. He was self-motivated and always profoundly involved in his specialist interests of politics and brass bands, the latter being the great love of his life – think Pete Postlethwaite's character in the film *Brassed Off*, and you have my dad. His name is Robert, but he is known at home as Brass Band Bob.

We have always thought Dad's behaviours were not typical, and in hindsight we can see that he is probably an undiagnosed autistic man, as he is relatively rigid in how he does things, always adhering to a routine. This was evident, too, in his social skills – or perceived lack of them: get him onto a topic he is interested in, and he can hold court about it. He always seemed to put his foot in it, to say the wrong thing. He never sugar-coats anything and can be pretty blunt, without realising its effect. While I was growing up I sometimes felt hurt by his teasing, which occasionally felt like shaming, but it wasn't intentional.

Mum and Dad's age at marriage was unremarkable, but their 'mixed' marriage was by no means the norm. At that time Enoch

Powell's voice could be heard loudly across Britain, sharing his intolerant beliefs about immigrants, fear-mongering that these people were taking jobs from British people and bringing disease into the country. Dad remembers his father complaining about immigrants, and when Grandma first met Mum she jokingly said, 'I was expecting you to arrive on an elephant!'

My parents defied convention, though, and any raised eyebrows, and set about creating their own family. Samantha, my older sister was born. Only a year and four days later, came my arrival. My birth story wasn't the greatest, either, and Mum haemorrhaging and being hospitalised around Samantha's first birthday must have been alarming. She had to have an emergency C-section, which back then meant the expectant mother was completely knocked out under a general anaesthetic. This meant that the initial bonding process did not happen for us, and that, coupled with me being a 'surprise', did not bode well for our relationship in the future, and it developed a fissure that widened as the years marched on. I always felt it; I just didn't know what it was.

As a nipper, my life was pretty eventful. There were gatherings most weekends as Mum was close to her siblings, so we spent a lot of time with that side of the family. However, Grandma visited us and sometimes stayed over; I loved it. She was only in Stalybridge, a few miles away, but we didn't have a car, so it felt like a trek to get to her, and so we wrote letters to her to keep in contact. Receiving a letter from her felt exciting. She was funny and smiled a lot. I think we amused her too, and she always had treats for us. I can smell her home even now, and I can recollect the quiet and calm atmosphere; everything was dusted and in its place, and Samantha and I would puncture that with our squealing desire to take turns using her old-style hoover, a Ewbank, on her already immaculate floors.

Like many people, my very early memories are accessed through family photos. It is difficult for me to recall anything tangible, like conversations and activities, back when I was small, but the images reveal our torn clothes, dirty knees, tights that were too long in the gusset, knee-high socks that fell from tired elastic that illustrate our humble beginnings, but also our big smiles. Mum and Dad did their best; they really had to graft to keep a roof over our heads, food in our bellies and clothes on our backs.

When I was a baby, we lived just behind Nan and Grandad's house on Manchester Road, a stone's throw from them, in a little row of terraces called Dalton Buildings. I love my grand-parents with all my heart, and I felt like they were there for me, and gave me my first experience of unconditional love. They always had a smile, a meal, wisdom and a cuddle for me. I had fun with them; Nana's voice was soothing, and Grandad enjoyed flexing his intelligence – testing us and teaching us, whether it be how to handle a deck of cards or teaching us about geography and history. He always let us look through his *Encyclopaedia Britannica* editions and challenged us on our use of the English language – but always playfully. If we asked, 'Can we have this?' or 'Can we have that?' he'd reply, 'I don't know if you can,' and make us change it to, 'Please may we have?' or 'May we do that?' God, I loved him so much.

Nana and Grandad were proud people who made the most of what they had, and we were always welcome. I loved their big stone terraced house. I can still feel the energy from my nana, and the nights we stayed over in her spare bedroom were bliss

– the religious imagery, soft lighting, the blankets and her openly demonstrated love created a warm space away from home that I relished. In the front room was a glass-fronted showcase with all Nana's trinkets, including a little model of the Taj Mahal. We could look at these things but not touch them. I loved staring at them – forever reminders of my roots in India. The back room was the kitchen that had a sofa, Grandad's armchair and a dining table in the middle. The adults would sit there smoking, drinking and talking for hours with large pans of rice and curry boiling away in the background. I would salivate at the prospect of the curries, rice, bread and pickled delights to come.

Although born in Britain, I have never felt English entirely. I have two cultural backgrounds in my DNA, and I felt it. Growing up around Anglo-Indians did not make me feel different to other people; I just did not see colour. Nana and Grandad only cooked Indian food, rarely eating English fare, and they were great cooks, so we were brought up eating curries and watching them being prepared. They are still the best curries I have ever tasted. Their delicious food filled my belly whilst my ears were full of their stories of 'back home'.

Mum and Dad were young parents trying to keep us all afloat. Mum ruled the roost, and what she said went. If ever we asked Dad for anything, even if we could have ice cream, it would be an emphatic 'Ask your mam.' While I did not experience the validation I craved as a child – no 'You are lovely, kind, clever, beautiful, talented, or a good girl.' I was well taken care of in a practical sense and I was grateful for all the things I had. I did not know what I was missing, as you don't know what you don't know about, but there was a void of cuddles and kind words that made me feel hollow, although what they did give me was their strong moral compass and a decent set of principles for life.

Everyone thought Samantha and I were twins because of our closeness in age, and Mum dressed us the same where possible. My mum made clothes for us and we often shared them. I don't remember the arrival of Stacy, my little sister, at all; she arrived when I was four. My sisters and I are varying shades of skin colour; Samantha is paler-skinned and more like the Sykes side; I have slightly yellow/olive skin, and Stacy is brown-skinned like Mum. The song 'Brown Girl in the Ring' by Boney M was sung to her regularly as a baby. It was her song.

At twenty-four years old, Mum was at the helm of a family with three little girls together – a tricky number – and all under five. As we grew, two would gang up on one in varying ways, and we would unanimously gang up on Mum when we were all scolded. Obedience was key in our house; you could not leave anything out of place and certainly never speak out of turn. Feelings of anger were not allowed, and conformity was queen. Mum could be spiky sometimes, and I learned early on not to bother Dad with anything.

Stories would spread like wildfire amongst our internal family, and gossip was shared with everyone, including stories about us kids. The first time I experienced feelings of shame was when I heard people speak about an incident when I was tiny and had been briefly left in a room alone with Samantha. She had pooed in her nappy and had taken it off. When Mum returned to the room, she found me with shit smeared around my face and all over my hands. Nobody spoke of how it happened but more of what I had done. I was a little baby, I was left unattended for a moment, I was exploring as a baby would, but it was used as a funny story to tell everybody, and the shame I felt was powerful.

Mum is a huge animal lover, so we had a cat called Snowy and many strays that she would let in, and even dogs that we would keep for a while until their owners would turn up. In the 1970s children could roam the streets, as could pet dogs. They were everywhere. I was bitten by a dog on the way to school, which gives me a glimmering fear of strange dogs even today, but I also love them. We did eventually buy a dog of our own called Snoopy. She became a massive part of the household but not always for good reasons. She was angry and pretty unhinged at times and could be aggressive randomly and fairly terrifying, but I did love her very much.

The Catholic Church featured sporadically in our life. Mum and Dad would go now and then when they could. Sitting still was hard for me, and trying not to get the giggles in quiet places is still problematic for me today. I have been known to laugh at completely inappropriate moments; later, when I was doing my radio show with Alan Carr, the producer Malcolm Prince would let me know if there was a sad email coming up because I would start to giggle if it was a tragic story and I hadn't been pre-warned. Obviously, it's not because I am a heartless bitch; I now realise it is very much a type of Tourette's that sits along-side my other 'conditions'. If people tell me their pet died, I can feel the creep of a smile on my face – I would even go as far as to describe it as an affliction. Pre-empting jokes was also a constant: laughing before a comedian said the punchline but not realising it was because I was a few steps ahead and knew where the gag was going, seemingly before everyone else.

This foresight has everything to do with my autistic nature. Where once I did not understand it, and it made me feel odd, now I see it as a great strength and have it with so many things. It is increasingly valuable to me and something I now perceive almost as magical. A sixth sense, a knowing.

Despite the restriction in church, I did love being in it. We always went to the church that Mum and Dad were married in – St Joseph's in top Mossley. It is a contemporary building, but I still loved the art, imagery, statues and smell. To this day, I always visit churches in all the countries and places I visit, and I light candles, pray, admire the arches, architecture and paintings and marvel at the stained-glass windows. I've spent many times reflecting on happiness in many pews worldwide. I am drawn to them.

Dad's love of brass bands was integral to our lives, and the Whit Friday walks were an exciting date in our calendar, which coincided with brass band contests held in Saddleworth, Oldham, Tameside and other towns around Greater Manchester. In a nutshell, these contests were, and still are, a big deal. The family would all get new clothes for the event – even new shoes. It felt so good to walk up to Mossley Brew to meet family and watch the procession go by – brass bands supporting different churches, rose queens, and retinues marching through the town with their bulbous, gold-tasselled banners towering above us as the bass drum kept time. There was an air of celebration, everybody was dressed up in their finest clothes and the good times were palpable. Waiting for Mossley St John's Band was the highlight – trying to get a good view at the front to catch a glimpse of Dad playing his euphonium and shouting out in support of him. It was thrilling.

Music is my second language, and brass band music is in my heart. I'm so proud of that bloodline, and the band's sound holds extreme sentimentality for my childhood and heritage. The brass band was such a big part of our family and Northern upbringing, it was inevitable that at some point we would all get involved, too, and later, when I was about eight or nine, Dad taught me to play a battered old trumpet that belonged to his father. I learned to read music relatively quickly, and got the hang of the fingering of the valves. I went to rehearsals sometimes, then later moved on to play the cornet as there isn't a trumpet in the brass band. Dad also taught Samantha the trombone, and eventually, Mum and Stacy the tenor horn. Slowly but surely he would draft us all in until we were all playing in a band called Ashtonian Brass and we were jokingly referred to as the Von Trapps.

I still love brass band music, and in recent years Dad and I have gone to the national finals at the Royal Albert Hall. We still sit and listen to twenty bands play the same music piece and take turns following the score, which is genuinely meditative, mindful and joyous.

All of these were special bonding moments that I've shared with Dad. Brass bands represent my dad, and they and he mean the world to me.

Chapter 2

When I turned five, we moved from Dalton Buildings to a new estate near 'Weldoms' where Dad worked, right at the bottom of our new road, which was positioned on Crown Hill, a street as steep as its name suggests. Our house had two bedrooms plus a box room, one bathroom and a garden at the front and back. I loved it and shared a room and a double bed with my sisters for many years. Their closeness was reassuring, such was my fear of the dark.

At the same time, I started infant school, just a short walk from the house. Often, on the way to school we dropped into John Robbies, our friendly neighbourhood newsagent, to spend 2p on halfpenny chews – fruit salads, blackjacks, flying saucers and bazooka bubble gum were our daily treat in tiny paper bags.

Mum was nervous about the roads, she would grab and drag us across by any means possible – clothes, arms, whatever it took to get us across without being flattened. Worried that we would get hurt, her nails would sometimes catch, and it all felt harsh to sensitive me. Apart from the roads, there was one more hurdle to clear. We had to walk past an animal pen, a large, fenced, triangular piece of land that housed ducks, geese and chickens. Often the geese escaped and hissed and chased us as we tried to pass. I would freeze with fear and hated their flapping, noise and threat. They terrified me.

I loved junior school, where creativity underpinned our learning. Threading beads, working with picture cards, loads of art stuff, trays of crayons, pencils and coloured paper were everywhere and at our disposal. I loved to draw and paint and enjoyed all the creativity that the setting allowed me to express. I always asked for Doodle Art for Christmas, having limitless patience and hyper-focus for staying within the intricate lines and the colour by numbers; oil painting sets – which were more difficult but none the less enjoyable – were always on my list too. I enjoyed the smell of the paint and the discipline.

I loved watching the television show *Painting with Nancy*, in which a lady with a dark, heavily backcombed bouffant hairstyle demonstrated how to paint with a palette knife and stood in front of an easel and talked through her process. I was engrossed as the final image emerged and the painting was completed. It was an adventure to watch its creation. *Take Hart* was another highly successful programme hosted by Tony Hart that I loved. I occasionally submitted pictures that never made the gallery, but it was fun to scan the line to see if mine had made the final edit, checking the screen with its famous theme tune.

The school assemblies were held in the hall, with its high ceiling and beautiful parquet polished flooring. Once a week we sat cross-legged in rows, patiently waiting for a television to be wheeled in on a long-legged structure, so it was up high enough for us all to get a decent view. Then, staring up at the small screen, we were treated to the TV show *Watch*, and we would shout 'Watch' when its title appeared on the screen. It was exciting and liberating to shout out inside the school hall, a behaviour that was normally saved for the playground.

I did not have a best friend at school; instead, my sisters were my playmates, and we always had each other to hang out with. With Stacy being that much smaller, she was our little doll. In fact, we once played hairdressers and we actually cut her hair. We completely butchered her locks and left her with a little scarecrow look, though with her cute-as-a-button face she looked even cuter afterwards, if that was possible. Then we took to each other's hair, creating crazy fringes that had to be grown out. Helicopter parenting was non-existent back then, which meant we had time and space to get up to all sorts of misdemeanours, not realising that what we were doing was naughty. I wasn't actually a 'naughty' girl, it's just that our mum could be a strong disciplinarian, and there were many house rules. She kept the place tidy and the sound of hoovering in the summer holidays was often my alarm call. I'm still an early riser today – who knows if it's nature or nurture. For the same reasons, lying-in simply wasn't an option either.

It was the seventies, and Mum and Dad were so young and had a good social life. The culture was that you worked hard in the week and partied at the weekend – a culture that still exists in this country today. Mum told me 'it was any excuse for a party', and house and dinner parties were de rigueur. It was fun to hear people arriving; we would run to the top of the stairs to see who the guests were. Coats were brought up and dumped on my parents' bed as more people kept on coming. Occasionally someone would check on us and bring us bags of crisps or goodies from the buffet until we conked out, exhausted from all the excitement, despite the music and chat coming through the floorboards.

One morning after a party, my sisters and I came downstairs to the mess remaining from the previous night. There were bottles of opened booze everywhere, half-drunk glasses of wine and ashtrays filled with cigarette butts. We went to town, eating the cake and leftover buffet food and tucking into the dregs of drink. Once finished, we started making the most hideous cocktails with whisky, vodka and whatever else was there. Stacy was only five and still had what we called her 'guggie' bottle that was usually for her milk, but it was now filled with a cocktail of spirits.

When Mum and Dad woke up, they had to deal with three very drunk and very sick children. I was rocking on the stairs asking for God's help when I wasn't running to the bathroom to be sick. It was carnage. We were all sick as dogs.

I don't remember being told off for this; instead, the story was spread throughout the family and amongst Mum and Dad's friends and we were shamed and relentlessly teased about it. When we visited Nan and Grandad, he would ask, 'What will you have to drink? Whisky? Gin?' We groaned with embarrassment for years to come. At the ripe old age of eight I accidentally had my first experience of being inebriated. But, of course, it would not be the last.

Entertaining at home was the norm – Mum and Dad even brewed their own when things got tight financially, so there were demijohns of brewing wine and beer in the kitchen that smelled of hops and fermenting yeast, an aroma that felt comforting. Every adult around us either drank or smoked – or both. Nobody had ever heard of passive smoking, and no one knew the risks, so as kids when we visited our grandparents we were shrouded in smoke for hours at a time.

At the weekend we spent a lot of time in the Woodend Club, a working men's club on Manchester Road. My cousins and I tore around the beer garden, never leaving the grounds, which were set right on the main road. Every now and again somebody would come and check on us, giving us the odd bottle of pop and packet of crisps here and there. Sometimes we were allowed to be in the tap room to play pool and darts, learning aiming games and skills that I have always loved. It was walking distance from Nan and Grandad's house, and we would walk home along the canal after an afternoon session.

The summers of the seventies were hot and long, and school holidays were endless weeks of play that stretched out. I loved those days running around the streets, with the kids in our neighbourhood, in and out of other people's gardens and paddling in the canal, fishing for tiddlers or pretending to be Charlie's Angels. We didn't need to go home to use the loo; instead we'd go wild and shit al fresco, wiping our arses with dock leaves.

My sisters and a neighbour, Julie, had a gang. We would create mysteries and become characters lost in our imagination around the derelict cotton mill at the back of our house. We called it going down to the cut; the deep hollow behind our homes that was a little scary and dangerous, littered with broken glass and probably a precarious skeletal structure, was our play-ground. We were out all day, only going home for meals, and we were safe. The only threat was 'flashers', which I luckily never saw, and once someone called the house to do some heavy breathing down the phone. My mum laughed so much that he ended up putting the phone down on her.

The streets were busy with people, and regular traders. The 'pop' man would arrive with the lorry full of fizzy drinks and we would beg Mum to get us a bottle of dandelion and burdock or sasparilla. Then the rag'n'bone man would come with his haunting cry, and people would load up all their unwanted items onto his cart. And, of course, the ice cream van was always a visitor to our street. We couldn't have one every time, and we couldn't always have what we wanted when we could, and it would be excruciating watching other people queue for lollies.

I also started to hang out with a girl called Wendy who lived on Cheshire Street at the bottom of our road. It was a row of terraced houses with ginnels among them – narrow passage-ways that I would always run past, scared someone would jump out. But it was also the flattest street around, which made it perfect for practising rollerskating, and that's how I started to talk to Wendy. Samantha and I shared the one set of adjustable rollerskates and took turns using them. I loved skating, always imagining they were ice skates. My first ever ambition was to be a figure skater, but for now I was a dirty-kneed girl trying to stay upright.

I was always up for an adventure, so when one of our babysitters who lived on the street asked if any of us kids wanted to go on the back of her boyfriend's motorbike for a ride down the road, I was the only one who said yes. I was not even ten years old, and I loved it. Unfortunately, as soon as I got on the bike I saw Samantha running home. She told Mum, who was fuming, and I was in deep shit and grounded for a week.

Wendy and I became fast friends for a while, even though she was a little older than me, and when I joined Wendy's Sunday School I got involved with some productions that they put on there. I have never been able to sing – I can hear a bum note from a million miles away, but my vocal cords aren't there in that capacity. So no solos for me. However, I loved rehearsals, dressing up, performing and being part of the production machine. 'Day Trip to Bangor' was one of the numbers in our variety show, and all the girls sat in a line as if we were in a cereal packing factory, all with rollers and hair nets, singing the lyrics, 'Didn't we have a luvverly time the day we went to Bangor, a beautiful day, we had lunch on the way.' Looking out onto the audience with the glare of the footlights, I stood up and declared, 'and all for under a pound, you know.' It got such a huge laugh, and I loved it.

I was an inquisitive soul and loved visiting homes to see how other people lived. I picked up their energy and little signals and vibes. I can feel soiled by someone's energy, as I'm a magnet with massive empathy levels. Growing up, my family noted my sensitivities because I was moved while even watching commercials, and I cried easily just by feeling everything. Happy or sad, I am still this way today. I am very in the moment of my experience and in tune with it. I allow my tears of joy and sadness to roll as I unmask. I believe it is good for me, and despite most people saying, 'Don't cry,' I need to hear the opposite. It is my processing and a much-needed survival tool for me, as it is for everyone.

The North West is known for its rain, but I only remember the endless hot summers when time was suspended and the long, dark, cold winters that crept through the woodwork of the windows and froze the glass. Four feet of snow dumped overnight on our little town with snowdrifts up to six feet would cut us off for a few days, here and there, meaning no school – heaven! Instead, we had days to build snowmen and have massive snowball fights on our street. We never had the right clothes for the weather and we wore socks over our shoes to give us a grip on the ice, and on our hands as gloves. We were sodden and frozen to the bone, but I loved how exhilarating it was to scream and be a little scared by the flying snowballs. Even the chilblains did not detract from the fun and the sense of release we enjoyed.

Indoors, I tried to hold myself together, being quiet and staying out of any line of fire. If Mum was upset with me about something, she would not speak to me for a while. Her silence was intense. I tried to get Mum onside again by asking her if there was anything I could do for her – making her a brew or offering to go to the shop were the only bargaining chips I had or could think of to curry favour.

I felt something was wrong between us and often wondered if I might not be Dad's child, such was my juvenile mind. Clearly I was my father's daughter, but with the disconnection between us, I wanted to understand why nothing seemed to add up. Although my Sykes genes were strong, I even thought I might have been adopted; making me anxious yet too fearful to ask.

We played when our parents were playful. Some Saturdays, when we were home alone with Dad, we played vinyl records on our record player and danced around the living room. Our parents' record collection was unusual, to say the least. We had a few Beatles singles, some from Cliff Richard and The Shadows and some old 45s, songs like 'la plume de ma tante', and we'd learn the lyrics of obscure recordings. There was an album of

TV theme tunes, which he would re-enact scenes for. The theme for *Black Beauty* would see us gallop around the living room as if we were on horses, and for *Match of the Day* we would pretend to play football. There were *Starsky and Hutch* and *Hawaii Five-0* to name a few. Dad would let us climb all over him, begging for a donkey ride or, even better, getting up on his shoulders without hitting our heads on the ceiling. I loved these mornings – carefree childhood fun using only our imagination, music, squeals, and rough and tumble with Dad.

The transition to Junior School was a giant leap for me. Every morning started with a quick-fire maths test and mental arithmetic with my headmaster, Mr Matthews. He was scary, to say the least, and my maths game was non-existent. Holding numbers in my head was an impossible task, and it still is. I don't know my times table even now. We had to pass our papers to our neighbour to mark, which was excruciating because five out of twenty was a regular score for me. The feelings of inadequacy would be set for the day. I felt out of my depth and stupid.

I don't recall ever not wanting to go to school, but I didn't really want to be there either. The school year was punctuated by assemblies where we would have to perform 'show' things, which scared me and made me cringe. We were all given lines to remember, but I was never picked for any lead roles, for which I was grateful. The panic of trying to remember a paragraph to say at the harvest festival was torture enough; my memory was never good at retaining lines, especially those that meant nothing to me, and standing in front of an audience like myself was painful. That trait never left me, emerging once again at the beginning of my TV career, though it was ignored by those I tried to share it with, and I'd find myself just having to muddle through.

I was always an average student; I just couldn't access things that the other children seemed to find easy. This was a trait of my education; I was never encouraged in areas I was good at and I had no clue about myself and my abilities. How can a child thrive in their life if the education system completely overlooks them? This was precisely how it felt; I was undermined, under-valued and unseen. From such a young age, I was so heavily masking, trying to look and behave like everyone else, that nobody could see my struggle.

Despite this, my life was relatively uneventful until my first experience of death when my Grandma died. It was a Whit Friday morning, and Mum got a call from Grandma's neighbour to say she had not picked up her milk bottle from the doorstep yet, and it was now late morning. Samantha and my dad were set to be marching that morning, and were already with the band, and Stacy and I had to go with my mum to Grandma's house. I saw her being carried out on a stretcher by the ambu-lance guys, covered, and I will never forget it. That afternoon we had to all travel to a family wedding in London, and because Mum and Dad couldn't do anything more for Grandma, we still went. At the wedding the next day, in my vulnerable state, and aged only ten, I developed a silly crush on the groom, and I would not leave him alone. I was relentlessly teased about this for years later and always felt great shame about. Now I realise it was just a direct response to my grandma dying. On the day of Grandma's funeral, when my parents came home after the burial, I heard my dad cry for the first time in my life, and my heart broke for him.

My mum and dad worked hard and had to roll with the punches. We lived in the North in the time of the Thatcher government. I remember at the top of the stairs, Mum and Dad had a *Jaws* film poster for years, which scared me, but it was eventually replaced by a parody of the *Gone with the Wind* poster, with Ronald Reagan as Rhett Butler carrying Thatcher as Scarlett O'Hara and the tagline: 'She promised to follow him to the ends of the Earth, and he promised to arrange it.' Somehow, nuclear destruction didn't bother me as much as being eaten by a shark.

The brutal realities of the seventies and eighties under Thatcher hit working-class people the most. One Saturday when we popped to Ashton-under-Lyne to get some bits, people were carrying buckets collecting money for the miners and their families who were starving just over the Pennines. We also were struggling and had no spare money, so clothes, books and toys were bought at jumble sales. I felt a little self-conscious about my second-hand clothes, but it had to be done. Power cuts were frequent, and we'd entertain ourselves by making animal shapes on the wall in the candlelight.

My dad and mum very political. Dad was always clued up about events in the world, opinionated and selective with his reading material, and he deemed *The Sun* newspaper nothing short of a 'comic'. I wish it were perceived as such by more people, as it would make it a less dangerous publication, but sadly many of its readers see everything they say as fact.

Dad ran in the local elections once as a Lib Dem candidate, once as a Labour candidate and once for the Green Party. He cares about the community he lives in and he speaks for the working man, having been a labourer for most of his life. He knows what he is talking about, too, and he has inspired me – his political stance is my own. He fought electoral reform – arguing for one man, one vote. He was a climate change activist before it was a 'thing', trying to recycle where possible, reusing old envelopes and so on, which I adopted very early on. I used to go canvassing with Dad – well, I'd post the leaflets at least. I was terrified of the growling dogs and hated putting my hand through the letter boxes, but liked the time spent with him walking and seeing a bit of the surrounding areas of our home.

When Dad was put on short time (when he was given fewer hours than the usual working week), Mum planned all the meals for the week so nothing would go to waste, and we bought a chest freezer so we could purchase a monthly shop and make everything last. She could pull off miraculous culinary feats with a few spices here and there and a ton of imagination. She made corned beef hash and cooked tinned Spam spiked with cloves in the oven – I devoured its pink salty deliciousness. My parents also decided to cultivate their own potato harvest, which was a triumph, and we also enjoyed a successful summer strawberry haul.

Mum is a great cook, and we were delighted with everything she made, from egg curry to lasagne. Her food was always delicious. I had an insatiable appetite, so sharing food with family was sometimes tricky. There was just enough to go around, and not much in the way of 'seconds', but Dad and I would hoover up any scraps that were ever left – the cartilage on bacon, fat from meat or the juices sucked out of chicken bones were the best bits. Very occasionally we would have pre-cooked food but mostly Mum cooked from scratch.

As well as my love of food, books were becoming huge in my life for the utter joy and escapism they brought me. We mostly borrowed books from our friend Julie down the road and from the library, or we bought from jumble sales. Buying new books felt decadent, but Mum was able to treat us every once in a while. The euphoria of being handed a new book and the intoxicating smell of the pages would make me heady and eager to get home and lose myself in it. I gorged on Enid Blyton's *Malory Towers*, *The Famous Five*, *The Secret Seven* and *The Magic Faraway Tree*. I craved the excitement, unlimited freedom and the children's 'lashings' of abundant fabulous food. I moved on, as I got a bit older, to Judy Bloom's *Are You There God? It's Me, Margaret*, which was talked about a lot by the girls in school. I finally got my hands on a copy from the library, and reading about a girl older than me going through puberty and its challenges was invaluable in helping me to feel seen and normal.

The last of baby me was abruptly over when my long hair finally came off. Mum was sick of brushing it to my yelps. I had a trip to the hairdressers and my new bob gave me a little maturity, and I liked it.

We loved the telly in our house. We had it on a lot, only blighted by running out of 50p pieces to put in its slot. Once the money for it ran out we had to wait until we got some more coins. When the box was emptied to pay for its rental, my eyes would pop at the pile of glistening 50p pieces that spewed out on the floor. So much fun to count and imagine what I would buy with it all.

My sisters and I loved the Saturday morning show *Swap Shop* hosted by Noel Edmonds, who was so wonderful and handsome, and much preferred it to *Tiswas*, the more wacky alternative that has never been me. As we got older, *Coronation Street* was a must, and to say I loved it is an understatement. The women in the show were memorable and funny and had all the best lines. I loved these women, but was a bit baffled by the blokes. Some things never change. We also loved Benny Hill and later Kenny Everett's video show, which was anarchic and sexy fun.

Seeing nakedness and how men responded to women was a turn-on for sure, and an eye-opener. The sexy dancers on *Top of the Pops* with their revealing outfits were just the norm, and titillation was rife on evening programming. One night we were watching David Lean's film *Ryan's Daughter* on telly, and during the scene where Rosy Ryan has sex for the first time with the mute soldier suffering from shellshock in the woods she started panting. I asked my parents why she was making that noise. Mum's response was to just pack us off to bed. 'Up the dancers,' Dad said, and that was that.

I wasn't yet ten, but I was curious and starting to have a sexual awakening, a tingling that I liked. I knew it felt nice, but I wasn't sure what it was and if it was expected, and I did not speak of it to anyone.

Chapter 3

Our childhood gang finally broke up after years of fun, and the impact it had on me was pivotal. I felt lost Julie and Samantha in one big hit, and suddenly I was lonely. I was getting into my teens, and my first bout of depression descended.

After years of the three of us sharing a bedroom, Mum asked if any of us wanted to take the spare room. Thankfully, there wasn't any arguing, as I was the only one to say yes. I was initially scared to sleep alone, having had my sisters so close all these years, but the thought of having my own room felt right. It was time to go for it. It took quite a few nights to get used to it, but eventually my room became my haven.

My musical taste was now being honed. *Top of the Pops* was a TV event that happened once a week. John Lennon's 'Imagine' was number one at Christmas, released as a tribute to him after he was killed. I felt hurt and confused when he died, and his message touched me deeply. The seventies and eighties were an epic time in music, and the New Romantic and slightly punky tunes were hitting the charts. I was into Adam and the Ants and worshipped Adam Ant, a total dreamboat and my first ever actual pin-up. I started to read *Smash Hits* magazine, pull out the posters, record the charts off the radio and learn the lyrics. My new bedroom walls were covered with his beautiful face. His 'Stand and Deliver' attire stared down at me, and my dreams were full of him. I practised kissing using my pillow and dreamt of the day I might have a handsome boyfriend or, better, meet Adam in the flesh.

Boy George and Culture Club eventually replaced him. George was hugely important in my life; I found him so beautiful. His first appearance on *Top of the Pops* had me and my friends debating whether he was a boy or a girl the next day at school. I was convinced and positive he was the latter and was shocked to discover I was wrong. I drew his face over and over and read everything I could get my hands on about him. I loved his beauty, attitude, his message, his voice and his humour. I collected all his press cuttings, and when I started to read about his addictions as the band's success snowballed, all the media criticism said what a bad example he was for his fans, but me, all I did was worry about him. I had his song 'Victims' on vinyl and would play it and cry and cry. His voice played havoc with my sensitive heart. I have never stopped loving George.

I was also obsessed with Lady Diana; when she came on the scene, I loved her. Her shyness reflected mine, and her youth and innocence spoke to me. I collected pictures of her and read everything about her, and she lifted my spirits whenever I saw her sweet face. Her unnecessary death hurts to this day. The way she was hunted is hard to forgive, something that is never to be forgotten.

I was getting older but not maturing like my contemporaries. I still needed help telling the time – Dad was still patiently trying to teach me, but the penny would not drop. I spent hours alone, filling my time with my books but, more critically, I was always thinking about how to survive the present. I felt invisible at home and desperately lonely. I learned to silently cry in my room and never show my frustration or anger. I didn't tell my parents of my pain, and they didn't ask after me either. All my emotions were in check in front of everybody. My nails were bitten down to the quick, and I twiddled my hair to soothe myself. I was unravelling. I started to hold my breath in my room, hoping I would pass out, with the sole purpose of being found. I had read somewhere that you could make yourself faint by holding your breath and squeezing your rib cage. I wondered if anyone would notice that I wasn't around. I never managed it, though, as I was too scared to take it to the end and pass out, but it was a habit I found hard to break.

My interests were many, and I seemed to focus on sports people specifically. During the Winter Olympics of 1984 and 1985, I was obsessed with Robin Cousins and Torvill and Dean. I would pretend to skate across the living room floor, gliding through a medal-winning routine, and I was absolutely able to take myself there fully in my mind. In my head, I was a champion ice skater, even though I didn't actually make it to an ice rink until I was in my forties, when the memory of my obsession returned to me as I took to the ice. All I can say is I did not fall or cling to the side. I was determined to brave it and totally embrace it. And I loved it.

I was into watching snooker and darts competitions on TV as well. If no one else wanted to watch it on the colour telly downstairs, I watched on the black and white portable telly Mum and Dad had in their bedroom; I knew where the balls were, so I didn't need the colour pictures. I watched these great characters do their thing. I loved Dennis Taylor, Hurricane Higgins and Cliff Thorburn – another of my juvenile crushes.

When I discovered tennis and Wimbledon, my whole world lit up. What a brilliant sporting event – being often set in blistering sunshine, it marked the start of summer for me. I was very shy and not sporty in real life at all. I hated PE at school because of the tiny little skirt we had to wear and the big knickers underneath; I hated the communal changing as I was so underdeveloped – me being the youngest – and my year group made it worse. I had no real access to tennis, but I dreamed of being a sportsperson.

The first player I saw was Virginia Wade; I learned the rules by watching her. I found a book at a jumble sale about the different shots and strategies that was written by Billie Jean King, and I could deeply understand the game even before holding a racket in my hand. I knew all the players and could imagine how it felt to play.

I adored it all – the crowds, the tradition, and the gentle cadence of the commentator Dan Maskell's voice. I raced home from school to watch the matches and I stayed up to watch the highlight shows, especially loving the fun montages of all the best bits of the day set to music. The characters back then were plenty; we had the precious Jimmy Connors, Martina Navratilova – just so good, relentlessly good. As I got into my mid-teens, 'Boom Boom' Boris Becker was throwing himself around the courts. I was just a year younger than him, and I worshipped him. I loved how exciting he was to watch; he'd never leave a shot not explored, he was so confident, so assertive. He was in a different class. My scrapbook was full of him. His Wimbledon win at seventeen profoundly impacted me and helped me believe anything was possible. I could not stop crying with joy.

Samantha seemed to be thriving. She played with the Mossley Hollins school band, appearing on the school album. She had a trip to Germany with the band, and her life seemed much more exciting than mine. I wished I was as gifted as her so I could make Mum and Dad as happy as Samantha was clearly making them. I didn't really see what my strengths were, or what my purpose was. I was a daydreamer and away with the fairies, only really engaging with stuff I was interested in privately.

Samantha was now working a Saturday job, and I also needed money. I felt too afraid to try to get a job out in the world, so Mum offered me a job helping to clean the house and doing all the washing and drying on a Saturday, for £3.50 a week. What an education this was. I wiped down all the skirting boards, hand-swept the stairs, cleaned the fridge and did the cupboards. Mum taught me everything. I was conscientious and good at it, loving the before and after look of the house. I especially enjoyed using the twin tub, washing and spinning the clothes. I learned quickly if I leant on it during the spin cycle it felt bloody good, and that became a bit of a habit.

The summer before I started secondary school, Mum and Dad had to claim some benefits to help with my uniform. I was wearing a hand-me-down jumper, the one Samantha had worn all of the previous year, and some ugly shoes that were bought with a government voucher. My skirt was too big and had hips in it that I did not fill. I had only turned eleven three weeks before starting secondary school, making me the youngest in the entire year. I felt unattractive and that set me apart. I had begun to feel conscious of my mixed-race background too. I wanted to be low-key, but those things made me stand out, and I hated them.

My Nana and Grandad sadly had to sell their Manchester Road house, the place of my childhood, and they moved to Micklehurst, to a council estate near the school, a place that was a bit more manageable now they were ageing. I went to spend lunchtime with them occasionally but wouldn't eat their curry because I didn't want to smell of it when I returned to school. Some boys had cottoned on to the fact I was mixed race, especially when my beautiful brown little sister arrived in the first year. I was called 'Paki' a few times and was picked on for being thin and flat-chested. God, I hated school. I was permanently on guard.

Outside of school I experienced racism only once, when my parents got me some tennis lessons at a local park, and every time I was practising volleys this lad would just keep calling me a Paki over the net. So I stopped going to tennis. The one big passion I had I gave up, because it hurt to be called names. It was best to retreat. I didn't tell anyone what had happened. I was constantly trying to be invisible, but at the same time I wanted to wear makeup like my friends. Contradictory as ever.

I was surviving my academic life and upholding brass banding with my family. Sometimes Dad would be conducting, but mostly he was playing. Samantha played solo trombone, and Mum and Stacy played the tenor horn. I played the baritone and craved the first baritone part, which Dad describes as the donkey of the band because it's a mix of everything. It was more interesting than the second baritone part of 'um chucks'.

We practised once a week; it was always a late night for us and sometimes it was very hard to be there. I was unsure of myself and didn't know how to engage with anyone. I could hide within the band's ranks, but I didn't know how to socialise. So during breaks I sat with Mum and listened to her conversations. If we weren't playing or marching, I just wanted to disappear.

At school, I became very close with a girl called Sarah. She was kind and gentle, and I felt comfortable around her. She lived in Carrbrook with her sister, Jenny. Her mum had left the marital home, so when we stayed over with her we had no parental guidance because her father was at work, and it felt great. We were free to laugh, talk about boys and listen to our favourite bands. I was obsessed with Duran Duran, and John Taylor was my idol.

At home I was described as 'the shy one', yet at school I was a 'chatterbox', and that was well documented in my school reports many times, even as far back as my junior school days. Some teachers I liked, some scared the living daylights out of me, and some were weak and let students run amok. I was easily swayed, so I would behave according to the social temperature of the room. I was by no means an angel, and I was a chameleon to boot.

I always enjoyed English but found Shakespeare problematic – too cryptic – and I hated poetry for the same reason. Some classes were just reading, and we students had to take turns reading sizeable passages. Some people's voices were a drone, no one bothered with intonation and expression, and listening to others reading badly made it even more difficult for me to absorb the plot.

I was always very skinny, me and Samantha both. People commented on our 'skinny legs' and 'bony bums' during childhood. Into my teens I was consumed with my body image because my body refused to change. It was straight up and down with zero curves. I was getting taller and was constantly aware that my breasts were not budding. I loathed my body because I felt it made me stand out. I was the odd one out; I never wore a bra at school, I didn't even have 'bee-stings', while all the other girls at school wore bras.

When I woke up to the blood and realised I had started my period, I was not ready for it, and I asked Mum for the day off school because I felt sick. She said okay, so I wrapped myself in a blanket and cried all day. I felt like every nerve was on the outside, and the loss of my childhood left me feeling exposed and freaked out. I was now a woman, yet I was still a total baby. My adulthood was knocking, and I was nowhere near ready. When Samantha got home from school I told her, and she told Mum. Some sanitary pads were bought, and that was that.

At this time, my mum was working for a company called Time Switch. They did the maintenance for the clocks within lampposts, which were timed to come on when necessary. Mum was reconditioning the time switches, and she asked if I would like to clean some at home to make some money. So trays of these things were brought to the house, and when I was overwhelmed by the volume everyone mucked in to help me shift them. They were black boxes made of Bakelite with a glass screen, filthy with dust and cobwebs. We dismantled them with screwdrivers and brushed out all the cobwebs and dust with small domestic paintbrushes. Some were worse than others, so we cleaned those with turpentine using old sheets made into rags. We spent hours breathing in the fumes while methodically polishing the cases and working the glass until they shined. How we slotted it in between homework, playing in the band, and all the other commitments that family life entailed, I do not know, but it was good to get some extra money. It was monotonous work, and the little production line in our kitchen was hard, cutting my hands to ribbons on the sharp sides of the casings, but I loved the 'before and after' element of the process, which for me was the reward and, of course, the cash.

Revision as a concept was a joke for me. No matter how many hours I tried to work and remember details, dates, places names, it did not go in. I could not store any information, I had zero memory bank. I just didn't know what was wrong with me; why couldn't I do it? My friends seemed to be managing it. After the career advisor visited the school, she concluded that hairdressing was my only option.

I had never contemplated this as a job and couldn't understand why she would think that it would be right for me, but I went ahead and applied. I was relieved to leave school, and thankful when they agreed, but it was an unremarkable end to my education. Unfortunately, my friend Sarah was off with appendicitis, so my time in secondary school dribbled to a close, lonely and without fanfare, and I never saw her again.

I had no idea what I truly wanted and no understanding of who I was. The youth training scheme in hairdressing paid £27.50 a week. I had never been outside of Mossley on my own and I was anxious. I was only fifteen, turning sixteen in August, and felt out of my depth.

My hairdressing career lasted less than a month. I hated travelling to the course; it was three days a week, then the rest of the time was spent at a salon making tea, washing hair and sweeping up. I was bored, at a loss around adults, and didn't want to be there. The sinks on a Friday were awash with men clocking off from factory jobs, steel wool matted in their hair; the smell of these metal shavings mixed with shampoo and sweat was nauseating and touching the men made me feel uncomfortable.

I asked Mum if it was okay if I applied to go to college to try to get my maths O level and do some A levels. I was not academic but I needed more time to grow up. Samantha was already at Ashton's sixth form, so I wanted to follow her there. Knowing that it meant Mum and Dad had to continue to support me financially for a more extended period, I was relieved and very grateful when they agreed. So I enrolled to do 2 A levels and try to get my maths O level. I picked Sociology and Religious Studies, not knowing why I chose those subjects. Why I didn't choose English is baffling to me now.

Sociology was interesting, but, again, I could not retain the information, and religious studies was not for me. Trying to break down the passages was laborious and too cryptic – worse than Shakespeare, if you can believe that. I was just biding my time, ironically hoping for some divine inspiration, waiting to grow up and start feeling like everyone else.

My social life had improved, and I went out on the weekends, drinking illegally for a while; started smoking and went to a local nightspot called Smokies – me and Samantha and our friends. Our weekly habit was dancing around our handbags to Luther Vandross, Mel and Kim and Terence Trent D'Arby.

I started to blossom. I was getting taller and developing – finally – and my face was changing. I was fixated on a boy at the college who I thought was really handsome. He was very popular and I knew some people he knew, so slowly I started to be in and around his circle. He was to become my first boyfriend. Luckily for me, he was experienced, so everything went smoothly. I lost my virginity to him, and it was fantastic, and that night I drew a rocket in my diary and wrote, 'We have lift-off.' Hardly cryptic if my parents were inclined to read it.

His father, however, disapproved. I'll never know whether it was because I was mixed race or working class, but he threatened to throw his son out if he continued to see me, which is precisely what happened. We were just kids, and it was really traumatic. He got a job and moved out, and suddenly we were forced to live a more adult life, a pressure that neither of us was even ready for. It was terrible, but we managed to push through. After that, they did not want to meet me, and I was never allowed to go to his house. So far, my first experience of falling in what I thought was love was not smooth, and my already low self-esteem took a hard knock. Mum was furious and called his father to challenge him. 'Is it because of her shade?' Mum asked, but he protested this notion in a way that Mum described as 'too much'.

Over the years, Mum had been an agent for Avon, Tupperware and a clothing company called Pippa Dee. Always finding new ways to earn a living, Mum would get a job during school, and then during the school holidays, when we were off, she would leave the job to be home for us. Being an agent for these brands meant work was manageable and flexible with three children. She was hosting one of these parties when some of the ladies asked me to try on the clothes for them, which became my first experience of 'modelling'. A colleague of my mum had suggested to her that I could be a model, which to me seemed like a strange suggestion. I did not see myself in those terms; once in a Domestic Science class I had been talking and the teacher said, 'Just because you are pretty does not mean you can get away with it.' It was the first time I had ever heard anybody say that, and it was confusing. I didn't understand what she was talking about. My self-esteem was non-existent; compliments were not part of the standard narrative of my life.

Despite being surprised by the suggestion of modelling, lacking any other inspiration for my future I ran with it, and Mum rang some model agents in Manchester. We spoke to an agency owned by Deborah Burns and were asked for some pictures. So a friend of Mum and Dad took some photos of me and we sent them in. When Debbie received them, she called me to come in and meet her in the flesh. Mum escorted me to the meeting; it was nerve-racking, but Debbie was kind and said, 'Get rid of the perm and the blue mascara, and we might have something.'

So that's what I did, and Dad took me to modelling classes at the agency on a Monday night in Manchester, where I 'learned' runway and a bit more about the business. I didn't enjoy it, I was so emotionally vulnerable and green, and my family and I were extending our geographical boundaries, which, for me, was scary. It was new for us all.

I did some test shots and was put on their new headshots poster. I was not a natural at all; I was incredibly wooden, I had no idea where and how to look or what to do with my arms and legs, and the photographer had to show me magazine tears to give me a clue. I couldn't fake a smile, either, and that was something I had to learn fast. Debbie changed my name to Melani Ann – 'Sykes' clearly wasn't sexy enough for a new young model. I was a bit miffed about the name change but I said nothing. Debbie put me straight on the books.

I was officially a gun for hire, about to become a professional fashion model, and I was terrified. I felt way out of my depth conversationally, my accent powerful and different from these city types, and thought I had nothing to say. Getting my 'book' together was required before I could start getting paid work. I did tests with photographers and tried to get some experience behind the camera.

After a bit of stop-and-start in the industry, I finally decided to brave it and fully give modelling a proper go. I started to work very quickly, and once you get some paid jobs, other photographers and clients begin to see you differently, generating more interest. So I didn't finish my second year of college.

My first trip abroad was with my mate, Kath. We gatecrashed a friend's 18–30 holiday in Ibiza for a long weekend, sneaking past the security guards every night. It was fun, quick, and my first flight, and it was an excellent and necessary test of travel before the trips began in full with work and I started to travel the world.

I was eighteen when I got my first long-haul work trip – a two-week calendar shoot in Africa. We were told that there would be a suggestion of our breasts but no nipple shots. I was a fashion model, after all. In *Vogue* magazine of late there had been full fashion spreads with semi-naked models wearing chiffon, and the shoot was sold to us in that vein. They had a glamour model to do the proper boobs-out pics, so I felt confident that what they said was true. I had to go into a room, chat with the photographer and show him my breasts. It was mortifying, but I did it. I could not look at him, just keeping my eyes on Debbie. I got the job. I was about to go on safari and travel through Africa on a steam train and have my first glimpse of the world, and I was excited – but racked with anxiety.

Everything felt daunting on the trip, but the other girls were wonderful and helped me relax. We stayed in a safari lodge, and I shared a hut with one of the girls. One day, I returned from shooting to find the most enormous bullfrog sitting on my mosquito net. I screamed and ran, and someone had to help remove it from the room. Unfortunately, my imagination ran wilder than the animals lurking in the black expanse outside. The only way I could sleep was by listening to music to drown out my thoughts and the sounds of the animals munching on the roof.

One night after dinner, when everyone had had a few drinks, the photographer asked if anyone wanted to have another one. Of course I said yes, but my roommate said no, so I was about to leave, not wanting to brave the walk back alone in the dark, when the photographer assured me that if I stayed for one more he would see me back safely later. We talked for a while and then, when we were wrapping up the evening, he said he didn't want to walk me home and that it was best if I stayed with him in his room. I was too scared to go back by myself and could not believe he was letting me down. But, he said, he was now nervous about dropping me and finding his way back alone. He was a few decades older than me, and I didn't think of the potential danger. I was very naive. He was the adult, and he knew it.

I got into the bed fully clothed and was worried that my roommate was alone, but I could do nothing. I was stuck. He got into bed too, and it was time to settle down. Slowly he inched his way over to me and started spooning me. I could feel his hard-on against my bottom, and now I was beginning to sweat. I wriggled away, but he moved forward. I could barely breathe and did nothing, just trying to move out until I was on the edge of the bed. I was very nervous; my tummy was starting to gripe, and I developed a dodgy stomach. The huts did not have loos, so I had to go out onto the front porch and shit in a bucket several times during the night. After that, he left me alone and fell asleep.

The next day, as soon as I woke, I returned to my hut. My roommate was not best pleased. She was scared and worried. I told her it wasn't what she was thinking, but I said nothing about what had happened. In fact, I buried the experience until recently, and it shocked me that I could act like nothing had happened. Still, I'm not surprised on reflection that he would pick me, the most unworldly of the pack, and I do believe it was a blessing that my body repelled the idea of him and saved me.

I was starting to get booked for lots of advertising and catalogue work, which paid quite well – Manchester models were being paid £200 a day for that kind of work. I was doing okay, slowly gaining confidence, and I could move better, have fun and relax enough to chat with people and make acquaintances. I was still fully involved with my home life and friends and was starting to enjoy mad weekends. The dance music club scene was massive up north, and I dabbled in it a little. We were experimenting with ecstasy, I had one terrifying acid trip, and I had the odd toke of a joint. I was now a full-on cigarette smoker and boozer at the weekend. In short, I was having fun – or at least thought I was.

I worked with a few London models who were paid to travel up to Manchester. They were put up in hotels, given travel expenses, paid for travel days and earned double what I was on. I could not stop thinking about how crazy it was. I wondered what London would be like, so I talked to Debbie about getting an agent in the capital. Their sister agency was 'Bookings', which was run by Pattie and Di, and it was a beautiful agency nestled in a gorgeous court in Notting Hill.

Mum helped arrange that I go down and stay with her auntie and uncle, Zia and Dougie, who lived in Wimbledon, so I could meet the agency and see if they liked me. They did, and I was put on their books. The plan was for me to spend a week doing 'go-sees', which are appointments to meet photographers, casting agents, potential clients and magazine fashion editors. I picked up work immediately, and photographers wanted to do 'tests' with me. It was a successful week, and the agency wanted me to move down entirely, but I was just not ready for it.

I started working with Jenny, a brilliant hairdresser based in Manchester who was beautiful, cool and fierce with a heart of gold. She cut my hair into a pixie style and made me look much more editorial for when I decided to brave my London career. But Jenny was also about to introduce me to another new part of my life.

Jenny was married to Jim, a saxophonist who had toured with the band Bros. We talked about Matt Goss, the lead singer, a few times, and even though the band were not aimed at my age group I admired his beauty and had a postage-stamp-sized pic of him near my headboard at home. The band were massive and on every TV show, everywhere, all the time. The posters in my bedroom had long gone, but this tiny picture I had cut out of a magazine was the last one standing.

One Saturday I got a call from Jenny on our house phone. Matt was in town; they were going out for dinner and could I come? Matt had seen a picture of me and liked the look of me. I had to decline; I was still with my boyfriend and we were going out that night. I was gutted, but it was the right thing to do. Less than an hour later my boyfriend rang me and cancelled our date, preferring to go out with his rugby mates. I was pissed off, and Mum said to call Jenny back and go to Manchester and meet Matt. So I did.

That afternoon I was a bag of nerves, but I got my shit together, got a cab and rocked up at Jenny's flat. Matt was humble, beautiful and shy, which made me feel relaxed. 'Do you do drugs?' He inquired. 'I will try anything once,' I said. I didn't really mean it, it just came out. Jenny dragged me to the loo to tell me Matt hated drugs, so 'don't say anything like that'. I shut that side of myself off, and we went for dinner.

The evening was fun despite my butterflies, as I listened to the stories about the tour. Matt was crazy gorgeous, and I felt a little out of my depth around him. I knocked my wine into his food, always clumsy, and I went to the men's loo instead of the women's, declaring to the table that it was odd that there was a unisex loo. I felt such a wally when they revealed to me I'd gone to the wrong one, bearings never being my strong point.

Matt offered to take me home. I explained it was pretty far away, a fifty-minute drive or so, but he insisted. He had a very low-slung white sports car that was really uncomfortable, which I couldn't help but mention. I got the sense that it wasn't received well. I am just not impressed by things, especially if they aren't comfortable. It's all very well looking good but is it functional?

The journey was lovely, and without the eyes of the others on us we could connect properly. We talked for a while outside Mum and Dad's house. He seemed shyer than me, so I heard myself say, 'Aren't you going to kiss me then?' He did. I honestly didn't know if I would ever see him again, so believe it or not I asked him for his autograph. He wrote secretly and told me to read it when I got inside. When I got to my bedroom, it read: 'Dearest Melanie, I hope I love you forever, Matt Goss'. I woke Mum to show it to her and tell her about the night. After that, Matt and I spoke most days on the phone, and he came to see me the following weekend.

Over the next few months we simply fell in love. I broke up with Jason, and when Matt asked me to move to London, I did. The day I left, I didn't go with a fanfare; I said goodbye to my parents, but I knew I would be home soon, so it wasn't too emotional.

Meeting him changed my life and brought me into an epic new period. It was unreal, confusing and painful. A child in a surreal, showbiz, adult world with no sense of self. A beautiful, loving, trusting, caring young woman/child entering into a crazy make-believe world with a new boyfriend and a demanding new city to conquer.

Chapter 4

Coming from the North West, London did scare me, but it was where my future was, and I knew I had to move for the long haul to explore my options. So I had to tough it out and deal with my overactive imagination and the capital's possible dangers. For me, using the underground was daunting; thinking I would get mugged or raped during the day was a deep concern and I had constant anxiety about the horrors potentially lurking around every corner. I had created a staunch and over-dramatised view before moving south, which I was trying to release myself from. I am always hyper-vigilant and sensitive while getting about, and I did not miss a trick; I used my keen senses and changed carriages when I felt unsafe. One day I caught a glimpse of a knife in the inside pocket of a man's over-coat, so I got out at the next stop and reported it to the first member of staff I could find, not being able to live with myself if I heard on the news of a stabbing later that day. I would shud-der at men's lascivious stares and slow approaches, jump up and scarper. A palpable lust directed at me would turn my stomach, which was a more common threat: low-level misogynists who literally saw each and every woman as a piece of meat, including me.

However, all that said, London was not as frightening as I'd predicted; my Gotham City-type notion shattered the more I found my feet. I was oblivious that strangers were the least of my worries, that the real predators weren't in that world, they were hiding in plain sight and closer to home, as energy vampires that would suck me dry and leave my mind and nerves jangling. I was so naïve, and it was a naïvety I did not understand until I finally got my recent diagnosis. I always see the good in people, understand their pain, and value theirs more than mine, which is a pattern of behaviour I have only recently absorbed for what it is. It's a dangerous cocktail of extreme empathy and lack of self-worth, which makes me a sitting duck for predatory narcissists.

One of the bonuses of London was its pace, which was quicker than back home, and it had the vibes that I enjoyed grooving with. I did not miss Mossley massively, yet I did try to get the train back regularly to go to clubs and hang out with my old friends from college, as I had a strong sense of love, loyalty and duty to see my friends and family.

Work kept me busy, too. I was getting a good combination of jobs: beauty, fashion, advertising and catalogue. I was a good all-rounder. Photographers regularly told me I was better in the flesh, which is a compliment but it is a bit of a shitter when your whole industry is based on what you look like in photos. My weight was permanently fluctuating. I was carrying puppy fat, never setting foot in a gym, eating shite and drinking too much wine whenever I could get away with it. I did a lot of beauty work and my face was my money-spinner, being by no means a body model. Even if I had had a 'good enough for the business' body, I was too self-conscious to show it. Occasionally I was required to stand on set in something skimpy, a heinous scenario I only had to endure a few times in my modelling career.

I rarely felt good even after being made up and having had my hair done, there were so many different versions of me that weren't me. I was just a 'face' to paint. It's understandable now why I looked better in person, because then I was more natural, and only a few photographers out of the hundreds I have worked with have captured that.

Despite this, I was managing to land beauty pages and some spreads in magazine, and catalogue work was aplenty. They were not as strict on being size 6 to 8, as their samples were for a more reasonable size 10, which was passable. I had to seriously diet to get to a size 8. But it wasn't just my body that was commented on. One photographer even told me I should get elocution lessons, clearly not used to having a northern girl in front of his lens. I thought it a ridiculous idea. What did it matter how I sounded? My voice wasn't required as a model anyway, so what was the point? Not least, I liked my voice. It's true it is in permanent flux, as I tend to mimic others around me and take on different inflexions, so some times it's softer than other times, but I thought the suggestion bizarre and quite frankly rude.

I bounced from sleeping in the model apartment in Ladbroke Grove, which was pretty run down and needed a new carpet and a lick of paint, and in Matt's uber-modern designer bachelor pad in Maida Vale. I was juggling a triple life; out of my depth in Matt's world, only feeling a connection when we were alone, which was rare. Time spent watching him write songs became extremely dull after a while – not because his ideas were not good, but because such is the repetitive nature of composing music. We played video games and not much else, and I was immersed in Matt's family dynamics, so much so that his life swamped mine. I never complained, though.

I was assuming a role back home in Mossley, too, playing down my life around my success and the stress that was in my work. It was better not to share it, and to just stay under the radar instead. I was drinking, smoking, swearing like a trooper with friends and being more myself with them. I didn't have the tools to under-stand that it was okay to feel all my emotions; I didn't need to separate them and go as far as to keep them under wraps, so I morphed into whatever everyone expected of me. How are you in all this was not a question I allowed myself to ask. I was just doing it, a chameleon. It was a highly skilled survival mechanism, but hazardous for self-knowledge and worth.

I had left Manchester amid the dance music scene and I was still pretty into it. Matt hated it; his love was soul and Stevie Wonder. It was just noise to him. Still, it felt good to let go and dance and lose myself in my music whenever I could. This phase would die eventually, and my love of rock music, guitars and lyrics would kick in the rest of the time and I developed an appreciation of music in all its magical forms. At one point I was obsessed with The Beatles' albums, lifestyles, messages and personalities. Lennon became a god to me. I devoured everything I could get my hands on about the group, even reading *Catcher in the Rye* because Mark Chapman had it on him when he shot Lennon. I wanted to understand the book's significance to John's assassination. This was just the way I was about everything – I would find a subject of interest and investigate it to its fullest, something that I still do now. I was constantly educating myself, a true autodidact.

Soon after we met, Matt and his brother, Luke, were close to bankruptcy after disgraceful mismanagement. They did an exclusive interview with Piers Morgan, a journalist masquerading as a friend who had encouraged them to bare their souls to the British public. People loved their demise, they became figures of fun, and it was relentless and horrifying; people spitting on Matt's car and asking him if they could lend him money was the general temperature of the male reaction to the news. Watching someone you love crash and burn and be tortured in the process was brutal to witness. I was only twenty and Matt was twenty-two, and I struggled to find the words to comfort him. I felt so useless and uncomfortable and very young. It was hard, but Bros then received an offer they could not refuse from John Reid, whose success with Elton and Queen is legendary. He had shown an interest in Matt and Luke with a view to getting them back on track with a third album. Later during the making of that album, John had asked me if Matt was interested in going solo. I shared it with Matt but what he did with that information, I never found out.

We were invited to Elton's birthday bash at his home. The driveway was a mile long and the house was grandiose and elegant. I was terrified of mingling with strangers and finding my voice with limited experience compared with these showbiz and music industry people. I started to drink to soften the edges of my anxiety; I listened to others talking – Chrissie Hynde commenting what a top 'lig' the party was was a word I needed Matt to translate. I slowly got pissed, argued with Matt, and lost him in the crowd. It was then that I stood there as a bystander looking into a world I could not access. I decided to try to get back to London. There was a line of black cabs outside the house; I had no money or chequebook. I asked the driver if he could take me back to Maida Vale. I didn't know where we were, but it was a trek to London. I asked the driver if I could send him a cheque in the post the next day, and he kindly agreed, and of course, I did.

I felt like a child around Matt. I didn't feel like a meek and mild person inside; I wanted to cut loose, be lairy and have fun. I wanted to laugh, have spontaneous sex and be free, but our lives were not like that. Matt was focused on his career and I just wanted to have a fun-loving relationship. He was a creature of habit and we weren't always on the same page. I would naturally put myself second; for example, Matt would prefer to seat me facing the wall when we went to restaurants so he had the view.

Over time, the relationship played havoc with my self-esteem. However, I found solace and fun with my friend Eloise. She was a Yorkshire girl, a model living in the agency flat in Ladbroke Grove. She was the only other London-based girl that was there. All the other models used the flat when flying in from all over the world; they stayed for a few nights here and there, never to be seen again. Eloise's Northernness and free spirit matched mine, and I loved her. We laughed a lot and beavered around London wherever possible. Still, we never had identical castings; looks-wise, we were polar opposites, her having beautiful flaxen hair and a different casting-call type than me. I needed and would have loved a companion on go-sees and castings on the long and often lonely days, but our schedules never collided.

Whenever I could, I went back to Ladbroke Grove in the evenings. I would go down to the corner shop, buy bottles of Mateus Rosé and Marlboro Lights, sit and compare our days, share stories of the people we had met and download our experiences. We talked about our castings and the photographers we'd met, our aspirations and our career dreams. We were coming up in the age of the supermodels; they were our inspiration.

I was attracted not to the fame but to how these girls could just command daft money and were looked after. The latter was something I so desperately needed. They were flown first class everywhere and shot by the most outstanding photographers in the world. They never had to go to castings, which was a real luxury that I knew would save my throbbing feet from pounding the pavements and escalators of the underground in search of work – this was as unglamorous as it sounds and took so much emotional energy. I would have given anything for that pressure to be taken away.

My work increased and I landed good jobs, covers and many catalogue trips. Magazines paid nothing; the images were merely currency for advertising campaigns that delivered big dough. You had to have good-quality tear sheets from magazine shoots in your portfolio to get prominent advertising, and the catalogue trips were financially somewhere in between. You also had to juggle the amount of catalogue you did so as not to be seen as a 'catalogue queen', which I personally had no problem with, as it was the only work I was genuinely comfortable doing. There was a set range of poses to show off the garments, and freedom in your body was required in an editorial, but I didn't have that. I was way too self-conscious, uncoordinated and clumsy to be that girl. A stint in Paris is also a must, and New York is to a degree too. I never braved East Coast USA, only visiting when Eloise moved there with her first husband a few years later.

Models had to be a certain height and dress size; it was a young woman's game. You also had to have naturally good skin as there was zero retouching at that time. You had to be bare-faced when doing your go-sees, too. Photographers worked with Polaroid film to test lighting, position and framing, then they moved to film – reels and reels of the stuff for just one shot. The photographer would not know if he had truly got it until he arrived back from the lab way after the shoot was over.

Anyone can now take pictures, alter bad lighting and retouch the model to get the perfect shot. Artistry has gone for many. The safety net of post-production makes the eye lazy, as I have noticed when I've worked with substandard photographers in recent years. With the old one-shot attitude, everyone on the team honed their skill set, not relying on being able to correct mistakes in 'post'.

We were allowed to state the types of jobs we would do and situations we did not want to deal with – like not wearing fur, which was one of mine, as well as no cat food adverts. (I have nothing against cats, though.) My other no-nos were tampon commercials, body shoots and working with male models – the latter were off limits mainly because I didn't want to make Matt jealous and I did not need the headache going to work and pretending that some Adonis was my love interest. Plus it was so just uncomfortable; I always found it hard to look into the eye of a crazy beautiful man, and the forced intimacy was excruciating.

My life with Matt was all over the place. His fans were only a couple of years younger than me and they followed him everywhere. For the first few months he kept me a secret, which did nothing for my self-esteem, but at the same time I didn't want to be in the limelight. It was bad enough being on the edges of it; people would fawn over Matt and muscle me out of the way or lean over me to get to him in restaurants for his autograph, literally elbowing me in my face, all while I was trying to eat my dinner. I could not believe how rude people were and how kind and accommodating he was, totally unaware of what it did to all around him.

Matt decided to get a dog for us both from Battersea Dog's Home; he just rocked up without consulting me, and as always I did not say anything. His name was Billy Ragga, and we adored this nervous, lovable little terrier-cross mongrel. The puppy training was non-existent, and when we returned to the flat Billy would have shat and pissed everywhere, having eaten half the window blinds and devoured our shoes. Matt should not have bought him; I was travelling and he was doing his thing, and eventually my mum took him when Matt moved to LA and keeping Billy was not viable.

Often when I walked Billy to the corner shop to get dinner or whatever, I would come back outside and there would be fans from all over the world taking photos of him. It was mental. Whenever we arrived home, Matt would spend an hour talking to the fans outside while I went upstairs; it felt shit.

While Billy was eating our shoes, we were eating crap. Matt's spotless kitchen with all the up-to-date appliances was never used. We always ate out and snacked, only getting a home-cooked meal from Matt's mum, Carol.

Matt didn't seem to have many celebrity friends, but we were invited to see Philip Schofield in *Joseph*, and his performance was a triumph. Matt invited him and his girlfriend Steph over to the flat one night. They seemed nice, but I felt nervous and out of my depth around them.

Being around him was not always easy either. The people around him, his 'team', had known him for years, and his brother and girlfriend Shirley would swing by for minutes, never stopping to hang out. But after the band's third album 'Bros' was over.

When Matt left the band and moved to LA, I stayed in the UK and moved in with Matt's mum Carol and her husband, Tony, for a while. In the evenings, we did crosswords and talked and watched TV. I loved them. They treated me like a family member and they were so good to me. I felt safe and loved.

Matt and Luke have a stepbrother, Adam, who is two weeks younger than me. He would appear now and again with his girlfriend and be at the occasional family dinner. We said hello but really did not connect much at the time – too many barriers and silent protocols and codes. But when Adam told me he was getting a motorbike, it excited me. Finally, it arrived, and I was up for us going for a spin. We had only been on the Old Kent Road for a short while and found ourselves behind a lorry. Adam decided to change lanes at speed, where we were surprisingly met by a parked car. I had put my visor down minutes before the crash because the wind was pummelling my face, so I had some protection when my face hit the back windscreen of the car. I woke up on the back of the parked vehicle, my leg trapped between the car and the bike and Adam standing roadside. I asked him, 'Are you okay?' He was white as a sheet and looked like a broken man. He thought he had killed me. Adam helped me from the car and the bike, and despite the horror I could not stop laughing. Hysterical shock setting in. We went back to Matt's mum Carol's, and then she took us to the hospital.

I was X-rayed and hadn't broken anything but I did suffer severe whiplash and a burn on my leg, and I developed a limp. I was due to visit LA to see Matt, but it had to be postponed. I have a high pain threshold, but the accident saw me retire to bed in Matt and Luke's childhood room as Carol cared for me. For a long time afterwards, I was a nervous passenger in taxis and would flinch at every bump in the road. Luckily, I lost the limp, but the PTSD would take time to iron itself out.

Chapter 5

Once I recovered from the crash I headed across the Atlantic to support Matt and have a holiday. I was twenty-one and this was my first trip to America. I had only seen LA in the movies, where films were made and movie stars lived. I wasn't impressed by that, but as a movie geek it was exciting. Their 'Have a nice day' attitude that some perceive as phoncy, I just loved. So used to the aggressive, unfriendly London life, it felt like a welcome change and much more me. The climate was also more to my liking. I always thrive in sunshine and heat; it recharges me completely and is my fuel. The sun's energy impacts me positively, and it's when I am at my best.

When I landed, Matt had ordered a stretch Lincoln to pick me up. I just didn't care for it. I acted happy, but it meant nothing to me. I knew he wanted me to be excited, so I performed, but really I was just pleased to see him. He was living in a beautiful place they call 'the valley', with a music producer he was working with. However, he was not in a great place emotionally, so I tried to be there for him as much as possible, and he tried to show me a good time.

It was exciting to be on Sunset Boulevard and go to Sunset Tattoo, the place where one of my rock idols, Guns N' Roses, had been for some of theirs. I opted for the tiniest tattoo in the shop, a strawberry, on my right hip, and Matt got an eagle on his arm. We went to see Aladdin at the Chinese Theatre, which was a treat, and seeing the Hollywood sign and clocking The Beverly Hills Hotel for the first time was fantastic. I loved the big outlet shops and vintage shopping at Melrose – and the two dollars to the pound was marvellous. I got a taste for Taco Bell and having to drive everywhere, too.

Matt and I were very different people, and many of our tastes were at odds; music for one, and his obsession with having trinkets and baubles that did nothing for me. All I craved was laughter and fun, not stuff. I could not give two fucks about diamonds, even though I appreciate their beauty. I do love beautiful cars, but these things are about craftsmanship, design and the view, not because they make good status symbols. I like what I like and I had never wanted stuff so people would see me differently, but purely because I wanted it.

Music studio life was incredibly boring for me; watching Matt write songs and sing would only hold my attention for a limited period. I'd already experienced a few years of it by this stage, and I didn't want to offend him, but the dark, airless caves where musicians create were not for me. I had to be able to see the sky, to breathe the air. I was not yet ingrained with my own will, so instead I sat being a dutiful girlfriend without caring for my wellbeing.

Matt was consumed by his work. I had come to LA so fired up and full of desire for him, then to finally be there only to find our expectations didn't match. It was frustrating and troubled me.

For the next year or so, I was bouncing back and forth across the pond. Finally, I got a model agent in LA too – I could not be dropping out of the game for nothing; I had to keep working. My London agency was pushing me.

The industry in LA was about health, beauty, advertising work and adverts. Cameron Diaz was a face at my agency, and the all-American blonde California girl was the hot ticket at the time, as well as the opposing heroin-chic look. I was neither. However, I did manage to land some work. It was varied, and I got meetings with top photographers like Peggy Sirota, but it was not the fashion mags that I picked up in the UK; it was commercials and a bit of catalogue.

A massive open casting call was held in town for Jean Paul Gaultier's AIDS charity catwalk show. Madonna would be the big draw, along with Billy Idol and the Red Hot Chili Peppers. Hundreds of people were waiting for the chance to be in the most talked-about event on the fashion calendar. The queue went around the entire building.

Finally, after hours of waiting, I was introduced to Jean Paul, and he asked me to walk for him. I am not a catwalk model and had never done a show of that size, but he gave me something to wear and asked me to walk once more. Somehow, I got the gig.

It was an extraordinary event. I was shy and overwhelmed, so I did what I always did – sit back, listen, and watch everyone else's behaviour. Everyone seemed so relaxed and comfortable, and my turmoil made me feel like an alien. To add insult to injury, I was told I would be wearing a blonde wig. For some reason all the brunettes had to be blonde and all the blondes had to be brunettes, which I didn't want, but I had no choice in it. One of my outfits was just avant-garde and awful; it was a straight-laced green trouser suit at the front and looked like an overgrown lawn at the back. I felt ugly and silly. While I was waiting to go on, Madonna brushed past wearing a pinstriped suit, looking so beautiful. None of us knew that moments later she would flash her fabulous boobs to the world, in the image that was splashed all over the papers the next day.

My agency was thrilled I got the gig, but I was unrecognisable so it wouldn't do my career one jot of good. It was, in fact, pointless – all I got from the experience was enduring yet another bizarre scene and traumatising myself in the process.

Even so, someone had come to the agency who had seen my card and liked my look, and I was surprised to be asked if I would like to screen test to be a presenter on MTV. This was a first for me. I was put in front of a camera, asked questions, then paired up with a guy I had to chat with, and that was it.

It was bizarre because I had never thought about doing television, so it was strange and a little exciting. It seemed to be a job that cared about what I had to say, not just my looks and body, and it seemed interesting.

I got down to the last few girls, but I was eventually told they had gone with someone else.

I was flip-flopping across the Atlantic to see Matt and the journey was becoming insignificant to me – once even going to LA for a long weekend. I was working in London but I was making trips all over the world and basically living out of a suitcase.

Catalogue jobs were plenty, and the drill was to do a casting, get the job, do a fitting, then try on the samples. It was usually three models trying the stuff on, and then we were allocated the outfits we looked best in for the spreads. Days on these trips started crazy early, often timed to catch the early morning light, with call times for hair and makeup at 3am onwards, before we even set off to the location. It was relentless.

People who believe that models' personalities don't come into the equation on shoots are wrong. No one, regardless of how beautiful they are, is picked to go on a trip for several weeks if they are not fun to be with. Auditioning for adverts was always nerve-racking, and the casting calls were usually huge, so you sometimes waited hours to be seen, which for me meant more time to stew and get into more of a state.

I was too shy to comfortably walk into rooms where there were lots of people, in particular staff from the agency and the director. You would walk in, then say your name, age and agency, show your profiles and that you had ten fingers, then they would ask you to act out a scenario without words. I never had castings that required me to speak lines. I was once asked to pretend I was on a swing, and I just couldn't do it; my mind could not get there. How the hell do you do that?! Needless to say, I didn't get that gig.

I did land some decent ads over the years, though, getting a Lucozade advert and one for Falmer Jeans. The filming for these required a bit of acting, and I was in every frame. The ad was reported in the *Sun* with a screen grab of me wearing stockings and suspenders, with the headline 'Matt Goss' girlfriend too sexy for TV', which was embarrassing and inaccurate as the ad was never intended for TV in the first place. I landed another ad for Pearl Drops toothpaste – after wearing red lips for the casting so my teeth looked super white – and I also landed a commercial directed by the great David Bailey for Barneys New York. I was excited to work with him; it was a catwalk scene with many models, men and women. After a few attempts of faking a catwalk show, he came onto the runway shouting at us all for not doing it right, then he looked at me and said, 'And you! You look like you're going to a fackin funeral.' I was mortified at the time, but it makes me laugh now because he was not far wrong.

Things were going well for me with work, and because I knew living with Carol and Tony was not a permanent solution to my homelessness I decided to rent a flat in Kensington. It was a small one-bedroom place with a hefty price tag that it wasn't worth because I was barely there, but I had to get a place for myself, some roots of my own.

Matt was anxious about our relationship from afar. When I was on work trips, he would ring my hotel room at crazy times to check up on me and I always had to share with other models, so he would disturb them too, and even though he knew this it wouldn't stop him calling. Often the model I shared with would get really pissed off at the constant disturbance and our arguments, so I'd find myself having to pacify them and him. It was a juggling act that I did not want.

I wasn't being unfaithful to Matt, but I *was* lying about my incessant drinking and smoking. I was barely in communication with my parents and would always cry and tell the people I was working with how lonely I was in my everyday life and how I didn't have good connections back home. Mum and I didn't speak very much; I don't think she knew where I was in the world at any given time. We just didn't keep in contact. I was anchorless and lost. I was bouncing around the world, seemingly having fun, and I was in a long-distance relationship that wasn't working and wasn't real. I always felt like I had to lie to him about who I really was, out of fear that he would break up with me if he knew the truth. I loved him; all I was trying to do was live my life.

It was weird to have a boyfriend that nobody met or knew. We would break up and get back together often. It was not a whole relationship; we were more like siblings. My role was that of a cheerleader and mascot for him, and I didn't want that.

My agency suggested it was time for me to go to Paris. That's where it is at in terms of fashion; getting French tear sheets and working with French photographers gave you the potential to land significant advertising campaigns, and the catwalk castings for French designers were hugely important, too. It's also where you might get spotted for *Vogue* and *Elle*. It was prestigious to spend time there and integral to being taken seriously as a fashion model, a supermodel, and being there gave bookers the signal that you meant business. My weight was permanently fluctuating – never fat, but sometimes getting a little too plump for the sample sizes, and I was five foot eight and a half, so on my model card it lied and said five foot nine, which was the minimum height requirement.

I was nervous about going to Paris, knowing it was another city to conquer. At first I stayed in little boutique hotels for a few weeks here and there. I could be called at any time for new castings or jobs, or new trips, and the unpredictability was always anxiety-inducing.

Paris was a completely different world, and I had to use my limited French – and try to expand it. I had to acclimatise to the Metro system, which had more stops than London. Following street maps and handling the surprises a new city throws up was testing; there were many homeless people and lots of people busking on the trains or just collecting money from carriage to carriage, and for me, one of the most surprising things was that some of the toilets in the cafés were just holes in the floor. I quickly learned to manage my handbag and clothes whilst straddling without accidentally peeing on my shoes.

I was lonely and relied heavily on my Discman for my companions; Nirvana, Guns N' Roses and Pearl Jam, Soundgarden and The Beatles were my musical chaperones. They pumped me up and gave me some semblance of confidence to pound the streets and bring some light to my long day's search for work.

It was in Paris that I learned how to be alone, and as hard as it was, I began to take myself out to lunch and sit in cafés on my own and be comfortable with it, with me. Paris was where I started to go to the cinema alone and live an independent existence. But of course it did not feel like that at the time; it felt like a necessity. But this time would come to pay me dividends for the future me, who would be alone and happy to be so.

The most-heard French word that was used to describe me by all who met me and looked at my book was '*tres mignon*', which means adorable or cute. I asked my agent what it meant and was told that I was a 'type', meaning I was a specific type – I am not Caucasian, and at the time and all through the 90s most models in advertising campaigns were white.

My 'mignonness' must have overridden my 'type' looks, though, as I found myself in work often, but for me the next hurdle was surviving shoots. The Parisians, understandably, only spoke French. So I couldn't really engage with people, and

I felt self-conscious that they were talking about me and I didn't know what was being said, but I started to read body language and the understanding of the words followed. I did pick up the language over the next few years and I always understood more than I was willing to speak.

Editorial modelling was more difficult for me because you had to be free and move well. You had to be confident, but I have always been clumsy and uncoordinated. I felt like a fairy elephant, a deer caught in the headlights – insert any other uncomfortable animal analogies here and you've got the picture.

I was also casting for shows and starving myself. The shows meant you had to be extremely skinny. I was running on cigarettes, a green salad for lunch (savouring every lettuce leaf) and a packet of peanuts at night. It was brutal but necessary if I was going to be skinny enough to bag the best shows. And when I was booked by Karl Lagerfeld while he was the designer for Chloe, my agency was thrilled.

Again, I was backstage at a huge show, mortified at having to get naked in front of throngs of people, hating my outfits and just feeling like an imposter. I sat alone and chain-smoked until it was my turn to walk, surrounded by supermodels – catching a glimpse of Christy Turlington, my favourite supermodel, was the only thing that made me smile. I stepped out with Kate Moss for one of the outfits and started down the runway to flashing lights, pumping music and the knowledge that this was one of the hottest tickets of Paris Fashion Week, so there were hundreds of people out there watching. I was overwhelmed and disorientated, and my only focus was not falling over. It was incredibly stressful, and I loathed it.

I was missing Matt, too, and our long-distance relationship was getting ridiculous, so together we decided that I would go out to LA, live there and make a proper go of it. I got rid of my rental flat and planned my move to America.

LA is not known for its fashion industry, so my London agency was not too enamoured with my decision. I was doing quite well in London and Paris, but needless to say I'd made up my mind and I went. Still, the agency had their eye on me from afar, pushing me to keep working, making sure I was living my life, not sacrificing it for Matt. I was so young, and their motherly instincts were unusual in the world of modelling. They really cared about their girls.

While I was out in LA I did come close to getting – and landed – what some might perceive as exciting work, but modelling jobs always held various degrees of anxiety for me, which is how I measured it. I was always on edge, never in my natural flow, but I saw no alternative routes at that time, so I kept marching ahead.

Matt, at this time, was stressed. His career and the album weren't moving along in the way he wanted. He never told me what was happening with the business side of things, so I was in the dark about everything, but it was clear that his future was uncertain. It was heavy for me to see him this way; I just held him and was as supportive as I could be while still so very young and inexperienced.

Matt was now living in the Hollywood Hills and had changed management. It was an old 1930s home with a beautiful view and no furniture – he had a futon in the living room and large empty rooms that needed to be made into a home. I was not a homemaker, and neither was he. We were kids. All the fixtures and fittings were old, and its atmosphere was quite heavy. Matt still hadn't released any music but his new manager was desperate to get him out there as 'the new George Michael'. He was talented enough, there were no two ways about it, and his voice is incredible, but getting him out there fully back in the public arena was an uphill battle.

We were invited to hang out with his new friends, but I had adopted the image of the quiet, adoring, conforming model girlfriend. I just could not find my voice around him. Finally, Matt introduced me to people who were more on my wavelength. We went for lunch with a music producer he was working with and his girlfriend from Yorkshire, Mandy. We had a riot with them. We had a boozy lunch, and it felt good to meet another Northern woman in LA, so we became good friends.

Matt's devotion to me had a question mark above it for many years. He said all the right things, but I was given signs while we were together that he was not being faithful. Yet I subconsciously chose to ignore them because I believed he was into the relationship like I was. Over the years, whatever the setting – whether we were holed up in a hotel or an apartment building – women were ringing him, even ringing the room. Once he went to see a woman outside while I waited inside, but still, I just believed him. It was crazy. I was in complete denial.

One day, I was home alone and opened up a phone bill, which I was casually looking through when I noticed many calls were made in the early hours of the morning. There were even a few that he was ringing a lot. I decided to check the answering machine, and I realised the tape had been removed. I suddenly felt the dread and realisation that he was hiding an utterly different world from me.

I was shaking as I rang Mandy in convulsions and asked her to come and get me. I needed to have a drink and to call these numbers to find out who these women were. The first person I called, I asked, 'Do you know Matt Goss?' She replied, 'Yeah, he's my boyfriend.' I could not believe it. Boyfriend! I told her I had been his girlfriend for the last five years. I wasn't angry with her; she had no idea I existed. I called a few other numbers, and all the women said they were 'seeing him'. I was dumbstruck, devastated and totally overwhelmed. I had been so worried about him being jealous of me, I couldn't believe that for all these years he had been, it seemed, prolifically unfaithful. I went to the bathroom and threw up.

I camped out at Mandy's for a while, only returning to the house to get some stuff a week or so later. The place looked a mess, like time had stopped. Matt was home when I arrived, and he said he was sorry and pleaded with me to forgive him. He asked me to go to Vegas to marry him, but all I kept thinking was I never wanted a marriage proposal to look like this. A man on his knees crying was not for me. I wasn't thinking about marriage at all anyway, it was not something I had ever fantasised about, but I never thought a proposal would look like this either.

I was adamant it was over, the trust was gone. Five long years of a stressful relationship had exhausted me, and trying to lasso it all back together seemed futile, but somehow I was talked into trying.

A few weeks later, my agency called me from London: 'You have been booked on a month's worth of catalogue trips.' I had been milked dry financially because I'd been helping Matt with his debts and taking out various temporary loans – ironically to pay off his telephone bills as well as to help him buy extravagant gifts for his brother, and I was broke. I needed the money big time. 'I'm coming home then,' I answered.

Matt and I were still together, but only just.

Chapter 6

I was signed up to two trips to Mallorca, back-to-back, with a bunch of new and incredible people, and I had lots of fun. The second trip was with a Northern team from Manchester, who were up for the hard work as well as the laughs. I had been away for a few weeks and was relaxed and ready to have fun. Being on my own was liberating – the drinking returned, and so did the cigarettes. Again, I was around Northern people who were fantastic, down-to-earth and kind.

I found the photographer's assistant gorgeous, and the feeling seemed to be mutual. His name was Gary, and he was from Doncaster. He was handsome, sweet, funny, creative and uncomplicated. He had a similar taste in music and introduced me to some new bands, like Suede and Oasis. Since being in the States I had missed so much English music culture, so he was filling me in on all that had passed me by.

I was still with Matt but I wasn't trying to appease him any more; my love for him had gone. My head was entirely turned by Gary. Matt was ringing my room, but I ignored his calls until one morning I knew I had to bite the bullet and tell him it was over. It was sad, the end of an era, but then, finally, after five years of my young adult life, I felt relieved and free from the shackles of a relationship that had eventually ended by phone.

Gary and I were totally vibing and having fun. I was coming back into my body and I fell in love with him – mainly because I credited him for saving me, believing then that I needed a man to catch me after a relationship collapse with another.

After the trip, I returned to London completely broke, without a bean. While waiting for my catalogue cheque, I borrowed £100 from my parents and was back at the model flat for a short while. I was starting over, but I knew it would be okay.

Again, though, I was now in a long-distance relationship with Gary, and with him up north and travelling, and me back in London there were a lot of phone calls and travelling so we could be together. I also had to return to Paris at my agency's request – just to give it one last shot. So I found a bedsit in Villiers in the 17th arrondissement, not too far from the Arc de Triomphe and my agency, to set down some roots and commit to my stay. I did love that poky flat, but in my gut I knew I would not be there for long.

Work was going okay. I secured French *Elle*, which was a bit of a coup, but on the big day of the shoot I had a massive spot on my face, and without the invention of retouching the team was a bit pissed off about it; no cover for me. There was no way around imperfections then; you had to be flawless. I also landed some good fashion spreads in *Madame Figaro* and a few fashion brochures for brands, but the extensive advertising campaigns still eluded me.

I was fed up with constantly travelling, with not being in London, and I was also tired of being alone. Gary came out to Paris once for a weekend, which was great fun, but mostly it was just me, on my own. I tried to get out and socialise, and I did meet a lovely model from my agency who invited me out one night with her partner and friends. We met at their apartment for drinks before going to a club. I noticed people were making trips to the bathroom at hers, and then I was offered a 'line', but I declined, happy with my wine. It was the first time I had met people who did cocaine. I thought nothing more about it, and we all headed out. I also met a French guy at my gym who was friends with Johnny Hallyday, and he invited me to one of Johnny's gigs; he could not believe I had never heard of him, such was his stardom in France, and he introduced me very briefly after the show.

Although my French was getting better, I still felt like an alien, and after a few months I rang my agent, Patti, in London to say I was tired of chasing the dream of being a hotshot fashion model and that I wanted to come home and just be a commercial model, do advertising, catalogues and stuff that meant I could be in London and not continue starving myself.

So that's what I did. I came home and moved into a friend's flat in Maida Vale, renting her spare room. Gary and I broke up – the distance between London and Manchester was daft and it just wasn't working – so I was back in London proper, and single. I was introduced to the London club scene. After being with a completely teetotal guy through my early twenties, and only ever really drinking when I wasn't with him, I started to dabble more and more in drugs, regularly taking ecstasy and cocaine and smoking weed. I even loved doing poppers. I generally became a complete and utter monster. I only did what I was given, never actually buying any, but the drugs were on tap. This new crowd I was in were all older than me, and I trusted them, but I was also heavily influenced by them, and they were all at it. I drowned out my inner compass and succumbed to being skilfully manipulated. I was abandoning myself and getting wrecked every weekend, losing lots of weight at first and then becoming bloated from the booze.

I was ensconced with the people on this scene and began a new relationship, which I knew was wrong, because he was older than me and with another partner. He gave me a sob story about his life and made it so easy to have the affair. I felt bad sometimes, but the drugs heavily skewed my sense of reality. I loved the rush and the high of the music; the dancing felt like a massive release, and the whole scene was addictive. It seemed like I was in a desperate situation but was being protected within it, too.

So when he left his partner without consulting me, my initial thought was, 'What did you do that for?' The relationship was supposed to be just a fantasy, not a reality. But instead of standing my ground and saying that out loud, I felt I had to go along with it. It was a terrible time in my life. The relationship soured, too – he was jealous and possessive, and then physically abusive. He would often get so angry, he would put his hands around my throat and habitually throw me against the wall. He abandoned me in vulnerable positions – I once had to make calls to get my agent to buy me a flight home when he left me stranded while we were on holiday.

My boyfriend charmed everyone. I had nobody to turn to and no one to share my fears with. He was going through a separation, running his business, and trying to keep control of me, and all the time he was untrusting and demanding. We were arguing all the time, and I was full of shame – I felt his treatment of me was punishment for the affair. I believed I deserved it. He played with my head constantly, sending me to a psychiatrist for my drinking. He told me I had a problem (which I did), but his constant plying me with cocaine meant my capacity to drink was high, and he loved to humiliate me. The psychiatrist asked me to write down why I thought I might be an alcoholic, and after our session he just said that he didn't think that was the case, I just needed to clean up my act a bit. I would be referred to this particular psychiatrist periodically over the next few decades, every time my life hit a downward turn.

I took the doctor's advice and started to slow down a bit on my partying and tried to focus on work despite all the trauma and temptation. I was still working and going for castings, then one day in 1996, while I was in Manchester on a catalogue job, I received a fax at the hotel from my agency. There was a casting for the new Boddingtons advert, for a new beer called Boddingtons Gold, which was brewed in Manchester and had framed its Northernness as its trademark.

The script was brilliant and hilarious. The recent series of adverts for the brand were award-winning and captured the nation's imagination, and had been spoofs on other commercial styles with a twist. They had gained lots of attention because they were brilliantly funny and they resonated with the public. The women who were featured in them were known as 'Boddingtons girls'. I was excited, as this script seemed made for me, and I instinctively knew that if I landed the gig it could change my career – but I had no idea in what capacity, nor what a colossal impact it would have on my life. I was sure this advert could be mine. There was no reason for it not to be.

The casting call in London was huge. The queue was massive – down the stairs and out onto the street. It was for models and actresses of all different looks, so I waited patiently for my turn. I hadn't been asked to deliver lines or speak to the camera since I had been back in LA, so I was nervous and excited.

Finally, my name was called and I entered the room. It was pretty busy with agency people, the casting director and the ad director, Daniel Kleinman. I did the usual name, profile and ten fingers routine, then Danny started to chat with me before I ran lines. The ad was a spoof of a Calvin Klein perfume advert; it was a stylish black and white film with a bunch of Adonises flexing their muscles, and I was a young beauty floating around – until I finally spoke. My line was: 'If you think that's a strong, chuck, try lifting one of these,' then I had to pretend to drink from a pint of Boddingtons.

When I did it, the whole room started to laugh.

'Where are you from?' Danny asked me.

'Greater Manchester,' I said.

They all looked pretty excited about that. Then they asked me to deliver the killer line: 'Aye, Torquil, your trollies ont' right way round?'

Again, more laughter.

I felt good about the read. Danny asked me to be Vera Duckworth on acid, and I pulled out the strongest accent I could muster, which was met with more laughter and a vibe of excitement in the room.

I left the casting buzzing and told my agent if I didn't get it I was satisfied that I could not have done any more, but I believed

I could very well have just nailed the gig. Waiting to see if I'd got a callback was painful, but finally my agent rang to say they wanted to see me again. After that, they called me back a third time. I started to think this was not a good sign; doesn't the client know already if they want me, and if not, how do they not know? Finally, I got the call. 'You got it!'

I was screaming with excitement; this was the most significant moment of my career. I rang my family. Boddingtons was my Dad's favourite beer at that time and I felt like I had just hit the jackpot, which I guess I had. Years later, I asked the ad agency guy, 'Why all the callbacks?' He told me, 'We knew as soon as we looked at you, you were the one, and then when we heard you we could not believe you were the real deal, so perfect for the role. We just thought there had to be something wrong with you.' Which made me laugh a lot.

l had fittings for a beautiful white, bias-cut gown, which was tailor-made for the advert, and after several fittings we were ready to take the production to LA. I was flown first class and travelled with the lady who held the 'purse' for the production. It was the first time I had been flown first class for work, and it felt great.

I noticed Gary Barlow was in the cabin with his lady and some music people. I thought maybe he was off to launch his solo career. One of the 'people', I later realised, was Simon Cowell, pre his global fame. Years later, he was a guest on my chat show, *Des and Mel*, and he confirmed that he had been on that plane. That flight had stuck in all our minds because someone fell ill en route, and the pilot announced he had to perform an emergency landing. None of us could have predicted what was ahead of us that day – it was unbelievable.

The first available place to land after crossing the Atlantic was Baffin Island, a sizeable Canadian island on the edge of the Arctic Circle. With its small runway and Inuit population, we must have been as much of a shock to them as being there was a shock to us. We were all dressed in summer clothes, ready to land in the sunshine state of California, and instead we exited the plane to snow and freezing temperatures. We were directed to an aeroplane hangar, where we were given blankets and some food. Nobody really knew what was going on and we were stuck there for many hours. We were told that one of the wings had been damaged on the landing, so we would have to wait for two smaller planes to arrive to take us to New York, from where we would try to get onward connecting flights. People started to venture out of the hangar to see where we were, and to check into a hotel if there was one and try to grab some food.

The 'purse' and I decided to venture out along with a guy we had got talking to who was a journalist. After a trek through the snow we ended up in a restaurant with the local Inuit people. The three of us decided to get a room at a hotel to sleep for a few hours until the first plane landed, which was for women and families. Finally, we were off to New York, where we would get a connecting flight to LA a day late.

I was completely nervous about doing the ad, and this crazy start to the trip did not help. I was always uncomfortable before any kind of work, as none of it came naturally to me, and this was the biggest thing I had ever done. I was so tired and scared I felt I couldn't deliver what they wanted and I had a bout of imposter syndrome that was crippling.

We shot the ad in Malibu, at a big oceanfront mansion previously used in an Arnold Schwarzenegger movie, I was told. I was introduced to the leading actor who played the character Torquil. I was crazy shy around him, I felt I might burn if I looked him in the eyes. The production was massive, with catering and even a Winnebago for me.

At that time I was reading a book about David Lean, the genius director who had become a significant interest of mine after I'd been introduced to *Brief Encounter*. I thought the film and story were so achingly beautiful that I had to watch more, devouring all of his movies. The lighting of his black and white films is legendary, so I was fascinated to explore the process he had with his director of photography (DOP). While I was on set waiting for one of my setups, I was reading my book when our DOP came over. He seemed surprised to see what I was reading and was curious about the book and my interest in it – after all, we were on the set of a black-and-white commercial. So we talked about lighting, movies and cinematography. I wondered later whether I had inspired or put pressure on him, but it was good to have the conversation and share our mutual appreciation of David Lean, and it really took the edge off my nerves.

In the end, the shoot went really well. As always, the build-up and the nerves went as soon as I got going. I knew from other ads I had done that I liked the collaboration and enjoyed the discipline of finding the right energy and executing it. It felt good to me, and I enjoyed my rapport with Danny, who is a brilliant director.

Before the advert was released, I was invited to take a look at it. There were a few different versions, but thankfully the one that went out was my favourite, too. A few months later it was released in cinemas and on television, and, again, the gag took everyone by surprise, becoming a smash hit.

After that, people started to recognise me in the street and everywhere; the advert was talked about a lot, and that's when the press began to be interested in who I was – and so did the TV companies. My modelling agent did not know what to do with all the requests. I did some interviews with the press, even agreeing to wear a gold bikini for a shoot with the *Sun*. I wasn't a body model, so I hated the experience, but, as always, I was going with the flow and taking advice from my elders and the 'professionals' around me. I didn't want to be famous; I just wanted more work. I wanted my modelling career to grow, but I had piqued the media's interest.

I was still with my boyfriend, who seemed to be taking my success in his stride, but the shit hit the fan one night when he hurt me one too many times, and as he was choking me I finally found the strength to get him off me and roar in his face for him to leave. To my surprise, he did. I took over the rental of our property and tried to keep myself together, but then one day I got home to the apartment and found he had taken everything except the sofa, presumably to sleep on, and a phone on the floor to harass me with messages and calls. Thankfully, I never saw him again. I was euphoric after he left but crushed at the same time. Why had I allowed him to subject me to that level of abuse? Why was I so weak to let these bullies into my life? I was so easily coerced and I kept getting into tight spots. I could see it, but even so, unbeknownst to me, a pattern for my relationships was emerging.

The Boddingtons ad kickstarted my TV career; I started getting some audition requests for television and landing roles here and there. My modelling agent did not understand contracts and advised me to get a television agent, because I was getting all the things I went for. It didn't seem to matter that I didn't know what I was doing. I auditioned at Sky to read the autocue and interview people, and I was offered a narration job on a video clip show called Reel TV UK. After that, I auditioned for MTV to do their chart show. For that audition I had to write a review, read it to the camera, interview one of the runners and read an autocue. I got that job too.

I was excited about the opportunity for a new career but I was sad to say goodbye to the life I had led for the past eight years. It was a huge adjustment; unbeknownst to me I was entering the lion's den, and I quickly discovered that the fashion industry had been a walk in the park compared to this dangerous beast of an industry.

Chapter 7

I loved my new-found freedom; my colossal screw-up and drug phase now seemed to be behind me, I was braving yet another restart and my new life lay ahead. Eloise was back in London, too, after her extensive travels and now divorced, and it was great to reconnect with her. We decided to rent a flat together in Chelsea, just off Sloane Square. I was in a new romantic relationship with a funny, posh, adorable and hilarious guy. Our class difference was apparent; he was from a background of great privilege that would overwhelm me now and again. Visiting his family pile in the country for the first time, arriving at the gates and driving up the gravel driveway, I burst into tears.

'What's wrong?' he asked.

'It's complicated,' I responded through my tears. I felt the gulf between our two backgrounds could be a problem.

But I was happy with him and my personal life seemed to be flourishing. I was travelling again and finding myself in tropical climes experiencing new things, finding new loves and interests

– like being on boats and fishing, and learning to dive to see the incredible reef. I was expanding my horizons and flying to remote corners of the world to find some peace, but whenever I was back home I was becoming extremely rattled by my professional life.

At first, being on TV was in some ways a relief because I finally had a voice and did not have to think about my body and how it looked as much, but there were elements of my new job that were difficult – I could not remember huge reams of lines, and I did not have the confidence to put things into my own words. Once the camera was in my face, I would go to pieces and panic would set in. I struggled with the earpiece, too; hearing someone in my ear would completely throw me at times, and I'd find myself answering the producer out loud instead of just quietly receiving the information. Working on TV played havoc with my sensitivities. I was not a natural, despite everyone telling me I was, and I felt I was juggling so much to do just one job. I knew my limitations and I would express them to the producers, but the people in the business kept saying, 'You are fine', 'It's okay', 'You are great', and all that bullshit. Nobody came up with tailor-made solutions for my specific sensibilities and issues.

I was being photographed, promoted and crowbarring myself and my personality to anything that fitted the brief. I was open-hearted and honest and spoke my truth in interviews with the press without understanding what the journalist would do with what I said. Everything got twisted and sensationalised. Everyone was shoving me in the direction that suited them – all the photoshoots for the men's magazines that were deemed essential for me to appear in required me to take off my clothes, and everyone asked me to do sexy shoots. It was insane; I had spent the last eight years declining work that required me to take my clothes off, and now here I was having to do precisely that to move forward in my new career.

I was being followed, manipulated and used without regard for my mental health. But wasn't I supposed to feel grateful? Wasn't this a golden opportunity? The reality was that now I had it, I just didn't want it. I did not want to be a sex symbol, a pin-up. I certainly didn't feel like one, but I did want to work, and my agent was steering me into all these things because that was the zeitgeist. I was told I needed to keep my profile high by doing magazines, and that in turn would get me TV work. Without it, they said, you are out of sight, out of mind. Of course, as I soon learned, agents also are mainly thinking about their 15 per cent cut for broadcasting gigs and 20 per cent for endorsement deals.

All of this took chunks out of my confidence, and I started to drink heavily. I was no longer doing drugs regularly, though – they had gone by the wayside and I only occasionally dabbled – as I could not engage in that world as I had before now I was in this new arena, especially with my growing fame. Everyone was at it, though. It was now 1997, and drugs were *everywhere*. However, I was determined that I would never fall down that hole again. No way.

I was working with MTV when I got a call to say that Boddingtons had been casting extensively for their new advert. They used a different Boddingtons girl every time because of the surprise element of the advert, but they just couldn't find the right person, and would I do another one? This time it was a spoof on a Nike advert, which was shot in Barstow, in

California. It was a no-brainer; I said yes. Again, the ad was a huge hit and further established me as a personality.

My agent got a meeting at a show called *The Big Breakfast*. Having not been living in the UK when it was launched, and being somebody who didn't watch TV (I preferred books and movies), I didn't really know the show, nor was I a particular fan of it or emotionally attached to it. Nevertheless, I knew it was a hit show and I made a concerted effort to watch it before attending the meeting. This was unusual for me – later in my career, agents would despair of me because when I met production companies I had no idea what kind of work they did. I was clueless. Not interested. I wasn't sure why it was essential to see their output because what was important for me was what I could do with them here and now. I wasn't good at blowing smoke up people's arses or 'schmoozing'. I still find it odd, and it is not in my nature; however, I learned that this industry loved it, and doing the research in advance gave me currency. Although it would become a currency that I did not want or care for.

The meeting went well and I was asked to do a screen test. They were looking for a showbiz reporter, so they sent me to a red carpet event to stand behind the rope and just grab people on their way in for a little chat. I hated it. I felt self-conscious; I had no mic technique, always expecting to know something before I learned it, and I had high expectations of myself and an imposter syndrome demon that haunted me. I got tongue-tied and hated calling out the names of famous people walking by. In short, it was excruciating. The thing is, I had either got that shit hidden or it didn't matter, because *The Big Breakfast* offered me a job.

I told the exec on the show that I didn't enjoy the screen test and wasn't sure if I wanted the job, but he assured me that the team would teach me everything I needed to know, and I would be fine. I was no longer modelling, this was my new life, and I had already made the leap. My agent assured me this was a big opportunity, so I signed the deal.

At the time, Johnny and Denise were the main presenters on *The Big Breakfast*, and Richard Orford was doing the subbing when the two of them were away. To begin with, I was asked to present the 'Find me a Model' competition, to introduce me to the viewers. *The Big Breakfast* was about to trawl the country for the next female and male supermodel, which is what they wanted me to front. The production team organised huge casting calls up and down the country for beautiful young boys and girls who aspired to the career I had just left to come and walk for us and tell us why they wanted to model. We had a panel of judges observe them and my job was to present the segment and be the conduit between the judges and contestants, basically to glue the whole thing together. I wasn't allowed an opinion on who I thought was good, though, and for the final they got Yasmin Le Bon to make the decision.

I started to feel like a puppet, yet I was always supposed to feel grateful for the opportunity. I found it frustrating, and I wasn't enjoying it. The whole thing made me anxious; I struggled to remember pieces to camera, and even once these segments were in the can I had other filming mountains to climb; I was asked to screen test with Richard so we could cover for Johnny and Denise when they were on holiday.

I was invited to the *Big Breakfast* house to do the trial in situ after they had been live on air that morning. I sat outside wringing my hands with nerves, watching and listening to all the banter between the crew and the production teams. Everyone seemed in their element and buzzing from that morning's broadcast and very pleased with themselves. Denise said hello, and Johnny came over to introduce himself. He asked me, 'What do you think of the house?' I looked at it and replied, 'It's very yellow.' His face was a picture. 'God,' I thought, 'he must think I am a complete airhead.' I sat there kicking myself as he walked away, feeling crushed and stupid, but I realise now I was just speaking my truth. To me, it just looked like a studio. It wasn't really a house, and the colour yellow was the most significant thing about it.

The test was challenging, proper seat of your pants stuff. I was holding myself together but I felt like I was totally shit. I was trying to feel happy and grateful to be there, but I loathed every moment of it. I was totally winging it and pretending I was having fun.

The production team was pleased with me, so I became the official showbiz reporter and stand-in for Denise. I was getting away with it, and people seemed to like me. As a roving reporter, I travelled and interviewed the great and the good, and the celebrity guests responded to me well; if any big stars felt edgy or pissed off, I could relax them and make them feel good just by being me, which felt rewarding. Some of the production team referred to me as their 'secret weapon', trusting me with the most challenging guests and interviews.

There was one star who had had a really bad experience with the British press for many years and he considered me a cog in that media wheel, and because of that he was rude and dismissive to me the three times we met. It was confusing, and it hurt, but of course he was right and was only trying to protect himself. Something I would learn to understand fully in the years to come.

One of my assignments for *The Big Breakfast* was flying out for the Oscars, which was really fun. I knew LA from my time living there, so there was no geographical transition needed, and with my ever-growing interest and love of film, I felt I was in the right place. Even so, red carpet events had my sensitivity levels on high alert and my confidence in pieces.

Behind the rope, we were crammed in with the press. Presenters from all over the world lined the entrance to the famous *Vanity Fair* party. When you're standing there you have to yell the film stars' names at the top of your voice, then if you bag one you'd better be ready. It was impossible to have watched all the films that had been nominated, and with my memory I was petrified of looking like a fool and saying the wrong thing.

One year I managed to get Julia Roberts just after her well-deserved win for *Erin Brockovich*. I had loved her forever, I was a huge fan of her work, but when I gently shook her hand and guided her a few inches towards the camera, she pulled her hand back and said loudly and sternly, 'Don't pull me!' I was shocked. One of the rope stands fell as I salvaged the 'chat', and as she turned her back and left, her boyfriend lifted the rope and apologised to me. The papers shamed me with a tiny piece, but nobody mentioned how an actress at the top of her game who had just won an Oscar could come up with so much surface anger to little me. I was stung and even now I can't watch her movies without thinking about it – though I do watch them, of course, because I still think she is a wonderful actress.

Cannes Film Festival was fun, too. The crew and I stayed in a little hotel in Juan-les-Pins just down the road from the city centre and the main drag, La Croisette. The junkets ad screenings were intense but I loved meeting people from all parts of the industry and talking about the films.

At the end of 1997, I did a shoot for *FHM* magazine for their January 1998 cover, which came out before Christmas, and was invited to their Christmas party. I took Eloise as my plus one to celebrate. The magazine editor introduced us to the showbiz reporter from the *Sun*, Andy Coulson, who invited us along to the newspaper's Christmas party at their HQ, which had live music and a revelrous throng. Andy had taken a shine to Eloise as soon as look at her, and they became an item after that night. I believe Eloise and Andy are still together. Unfortunately for me, hanging around a showbiz journalist wasn't just dangerous but highly uncomfortable. How could I possibly drop my guard around this man? Unfortunately, Eloise moved out of our flat and I slowly lost contact with her after nearly ten years of friendship. It broke my heart but I had to walk away, I just didn't trust him.

My boyfriend and I were still going strong and we decided to get a place together in Notting Hill. It was to be pleasure and pain, as we didn't last very long after that. We partied too much, and the relationship wasn't working for me. The irony was that I got much worse after I asked him to leave. My mental health wasn't good, and adapting to my new-found fame was hurting me. I was young, too famous for comfort, drinking too much for my health and being manipulated externally at every turn. The press watched my every move, blowing up stories and trying to shame me. The whole 'Ladette' label they had created was a joke

– I drank pints so I didn't have to go to the bar as much; I certainly wasn't trying to match the lads. It's not who I am, and I don't do things for effect, either. What you see is who I am.

I was out of my depth in groups of people, preferring to get silly with a select few. Some of these were strangers that I let into my home, and I trusted people who did not care about me. I was not in my body, I had no sense of self, and I was clearly damaged. I had lost my self-respect, getting home drunk every night and not even securing my home. I woke up most days with dreadful emotional and physical hangovers, feeling full of shame and anger at myself. But I got myself out of bed, put my house in order, showered and swept all my feelings of disgust under the carpet and went again. While I was at an all-time low, I was seriously depressed but masquerading as fun me. I just couldn't slow myself down enough to deal with it. The only person that talked to me about it was Mark Wogan, my sole sober friend. He suggested I might be depressed and that I should see a doctor and take some antidepressants, but I was in deep denial. Everyone else was along for the ride, while protecting themselves but not me. I would seek out people to get drunk with and just keep pressing that 'fuck it' button. I had no love for myself at all. It was quite a dark time.

I don't know how my fame affected my family, as I didn't share my pain with them and I played down my success. I rarely went home, only communicating with the odd phone call to my sisters and parents and my Nan and Grandad. Mum visited London quite a few times to meet my friends and see how I was living, and I held it together enough to give her the impression that I wasn't wholly unravelling despite my drinking every day.

I had my agent, Amanda, who took care of me and my business; we were all young and stupid, and nobody was in their bodies. Luckily there weren't any social media channels back then, and no one had camera phones, so at least I had some semblance of privacy – or so I thought. I often wondered how the paps knew where I was, and how they got hold of the news stories that covered private matters I hadn't shared publicly.

People perceive the fashion world to be bitchy, but I found the entertainment industry sphere next-level cutthroat and toxic. Hilariously, people would say to me, 'I bet you're glad you're out of the fashion industry,' but the constant press attention that stemmed from my TV profile was killing me. I was always being written up in a misogynistic way, being shamed and exposed for my 'behaviour' and branded 'Maneater Mel', as if I was some kind of predator, which is just not me. Every famous man I was photographed with or seen with at that time was written up as a lover. Some stories were literally made up and others were warped beyond recognition. In recent years I have heartbreakingly discovered that I was being phone-hacked by the tabloids between 1997 and 2010. And all because a picture of me or a story about my life sold papers.

I was just a twenty-something trying to work out who I was and living my life, which included finding love and having a sex life. I was trying to have fun with people, make friends, enjoy good food, conversation and travel, but against a backdrop of slut-shaming, heartache and fear. Nobody gave a fuck about my mental health. Nothing was sacred in my life; I was a commodity to make money and used to feed the public – who the tabloid press looked down upon and condescended – with morsels of salacious, debased and distorted versions of the truth. They still do.

Though many of the stories were pure lies, there was nothing I could do about it. The channels and production companies you work with do not help you with the fallout of fame, which was brutal. The narrative is that you are paid well so you must endure the crap that goes with it. Which is nonsense. Yes, you are paid well (though the figures in the press were highly inflated and not accurate), but everyone else's profit is off the chart, and they take none of the heat. As far as I am concerned, the fee is for the work and what you bring to the company, which is eyeballs – the public. A presenter's role is to be the bait to lure in the viewers and raise those all-important ratings. Getting down to brass tacks, I understood that was what I was paid for, certainly not danger money, and if that is what it's about, it is not nearly enough.

It was a crazy time. My profile was sky-high for all the wrong reasons, but I was still being offered decent work. I landed a radio show called *TFI on Galaxy*, Galaxy being a country-wide commercial radio station that had secured the rights to access *TFI Friday*, the successful weekly Channel 4 chat show that had Chris Evans at the helm. I was booked to conduct audio-only interviews with all his guests.

From the get-go of my new career, interviewing people was my forte. I could put people at ease and so they opened up to me; I loved that element of the job, and still do. Doing my research by reading authors' books, watching someone's movie, exploring creative people's work and talking about their processes was such a buzz. I love artists in any field, so the actual work was good, and the pressure was off to a degree because I had no cameras stuck in my face. I learned quickly that the radio was my favourite thing to do – I no longer felt I had to take a leap to be 'me'; I could just be me.

TFI was anarchic, uproarious fun. I never drank before work; I was disciplined only because I was too paranoid for that; however, afterwards it was a different story; everyone got leathered. We piled over to the pub across the road from the studio and drank. Chris, the crew and all the guests were out for the night, and it was mental. My radio show was live every Saturday morning, so I was always hungover for it. I was a high-functioning drinker at this point, surrounded by many in a similar position, Chris being one of them. I could still get my shit together, get to work and give an acceptable performance.

After a few weeks on the job I became totally enamoured with Chris. He was confident, funny and intelligent, I was starry-eyed for him and I fell for him. What a disaster. The feelings were not reciprocated, but we spent some daft times together, and although he wasn't harmful to me he wasn't particularly nice to me either. Mostly, we were just steaming drunk.

I was turning down work and not doing everything that was offered to me. There was so much shit being made for television that I wasn't interested in being part of, and some of the roles were just lame. I avoided live TV wherever possible because it terrified me; I was often throwing up with nerves in the loo before *The Big Breakfast* and having sleepless nights ahead of the shows.

I have always had an instinct for what is right for me work-wise and I go off that path at my peril, but even so I was in varying degrees of discomfort all the time. I was kidding myself that I was brave and should do what scared me, but by doing this I was stringing myself out emotionally. Television just wasn't the profession for me, and the circus around it was killing me, but at that time I felt I had no other choices. I was hypersensitive, and the drinking was taking the edge off everything. I was drinking to celebrate, commiserate and endure all interactions with people in every area of my life, public and private.

During these heady days, I bumped into Matt. I was leaving Harvey Nichols when I heard someone shout 'Melly'. The only person who called me that (except my nieces and nephews, who call me Auntie Melly) was him. I turned around and there he was, in the flesh in London. We had not seen or spoken to each other for three years, and so much had changed in that time, but it was good to see him. I found myself hanging out with him again, and he started to tell the press that we used to be an item. I hadn't mentioned it to the media at all, because I felt it was nobody's business and I didn't think it relevant, but here he was letting everyone know, and I was a little miffed.

Matt introduced me to his friend Max Beesley during one of our lunches. I liked him; he was funny, sexy and Northern. I first got talking to Max about acting, as I had enjoyed my relationship with most directors thus far and thought it would be an interesting avenue to explore. He steered me towards Sheila Gray, a method acting coach in New York. I enrolled in and flew out for a two-week course, in which I experienced some immersive therapy and acting classes. My reliance on alcohol came up in one of these sessions, and as a result I went to my first ever AA meeting. The whole thing was fascinating. Still, I wasn't ready for it in any way, shape or form. In terms of the acting, the upshot of the whole trip was that improvisation was my forte, I could be given a character breakdown and act it out, and because nobody knew who I was I felt able to be vulnerable and freer.

But my memory was still awful and I could see that remembering lines would always be problematic. I loved improv, but it was clear that neither Ken Loach nor Mike Leigh would be knocking on my door any time soon.

My relationship with Max had developed into a love match, but it wasn't to be. Despite our crazy chemistry, we were on entirely different plains. There were tonnes of press stories around that relationship, and the interest in us was huge, but unfortunately he wasn't happy, and neither was I. However, Max did get me into football. He took me to an FA Cup Final in 1999 and we watched Manchester Utd clinch the title against Newcastle. This gateway to my love of football made me a firm Manchester United fan from then on. Max and I both made some daft decisions in the relationship, and soon it was over. Silver linings, though: my love for football and my knowledge of the game have grown over the decades, and Max and I are still good friends.

Christmas was looming, so I decided to escape to Jamaica for Christmas and New Year alone. I cried, mourned, went on a fishing trip and caught three bonito tuna on an excursion out to sea – always a lucky fisherwoman – read a lot of books, got attached to an American couple that were holidaying there too and tried to heal once again. But I was so troubled; another relationship had hit the dust. I was at an all-time low.

My biological clock was ticking loud for the first time in my life; I wanted to settle down, but I wasn't in any fit state to. I was drinking heavily – nightly – occasionally trying to slow down, but only managing three days tops without succumbing to its medicinal pull. I was treating people to nights outs and dinners, constantly feeling obligated to foot the bill for everyone. And of course everyone accepted the offer. Why wouldn't they? If I wanted to go on holiday, I paid for people so I didn't always have to go alone.

I was experiencing a lot of emotional suffering, too, getting sexually involved with people I wasn't really into, without any regard for myself, and feeling a desolation I'd never known before. My relationship with my mum was damaged when she was doorstepped by the *News of the World*. The journalists had knocked on her door and said they were from *Hello* magazine. She told me she had felt bamboozled into opening my childhood home to them, and letting them take pics of her and giving access to family photographs. I was livid and annoyed for a very long time. The press intrusion was so great; I could not believe that they had got into my childhood home.

Then I met Daniel. Daniel Caltagirone was an actor who had just starred in a Channel 4 TV series called *Lock Stock*, which was produced by Guy Ritchie off the back of the success of the film *Lock Stock and Two Smoking Barrels*. Daniel played one of the leads, and while he was doing the press rounds he was booked onto my Galaxy radio show. When he arrived, I was bent over the nearly empty water cooler, desperately trying to eke out the remains to quench my raging hangover thirst, and he walked in behind me. I turned around to greet him. He was suited and booted and dressed for the races, where he was heading after the show. He looked sharp and handsome, and he was utterly charming. He flirted with me on air and even asked me to go away with him during the broadcast. I liked him a lot. I was about to turn thirty, in denial about my drinking, chain-smoking like there was no tomorrow, in a career that I didn't realise was killing me and all in all pretty miserable. Still, suddenly I felt excited about him. But he was not going to put up with my bullshit, and he was not going to leave me alone either.

Chapter 8

Daniel is a second-generation Sicilian, fluent in Italian, an exceptional cook and charming to a fault. He felt exotic to me, a cut above the rest. He seemed smart, funny and like nobody I had met before; it was a whole new experience. I fell for him even though, just like Matt, his need to do things his way was entrenched from the get-go, so subtle at first that I did not see it, or, to be more accurate, I didn't want to. This was what love looked like; I did not know any different.

Daniel was hours late for our first date — one of his traits that never waned and permanently left me rankled. I was the opposite; I was always on time, always punctual and professional to a fault in my work life and across all my domestic and personal commitments. I never left a bill unpaid, a cushion not plumped — my flat was pristine — and still managing to permanently have a book on the go. All the mechanics of my life were a well-oiled machine, which was totally at odds with my mental state. I was high functioning yet my inner world was marred with chaos.

Alcohol was my weakness. I was incredibly drunk when Daniel arrived to take me out on our second date. It was a Sunday and I'd been drinking pints with tequila chasers at the local pub all afternoon. Yep, I know. It was Dutch courage that turned into me abandoning myself altogether and pressing the 'fuck it' button once again, the 'I can do what I want' attitude. Hell, I did not believe I deserved love anyway.

My drinking was, at that time, a confidence booster, a way to brave the world and calm my ragged nerves, and my tolerance for alcohol was high. I never wanted to be alone, or home alone, and I absolutely hated my own company – I would even go to the pub to read a book. Having a few drinks relaxed me, then adopting a devil-may-care attitude would descend, and more drinks would follow. The pattern was there, I just wasn't aware of it. I was in no shape to be taken out for dinner, and he made it very clear that this behaviour was unacceptable and that I needed help. At first I argued with him. Who the fuck was this guy to come into my life for five minutes and tell me what to do? I wanted him to go, to leave me to it. I was so sick of men trying to control me, but he would not give up. He encouraged me to get a psychiatrist, get a diagnosis and finally get my shit together. Despite my temerity and defence of my behaviour, I broke; I was terrified of losing him, so I agreed to his plan of action.

His concern for me I read as a loving act, which I'm sure it was, but partly I also read it as control. Daniel asked about my past, and I told him as much as I thought he could handle, but he hated all of it. He questioned me on details of my past relationships and who I had been with. I had to break down news stories he had read about me to scrape away the lies, unpick them and get to the truth, all to stop him worrying. It was a painful practice. I barely asked about his past; for one, I didn't care what came before me, what was important was now, and two, I wanted to demonstrate the type of relationship I wanted to be in. I had been with a few jealous, possessive men in the past, so there was no space for any insecurity in me. I always felt I must lead by example, but it never worked. To assuage his worries, I felt I had to restrict who I spoke to and had in my life, even stopping seeing one of my best male friends.

I was referred to the same psychiatrist I had met back in my clubbing days, who put me on antidepressants and referred me to a therapist. In the sessions, I revealed my thoughts about my childhood for the first time, and talked about my early feelings of being lonely and rudderless. We discussed that I had been a depressive from an early age, possibly pre-dating my teens, and it all started to make a little more sense. It hadn't been in my imagination; I was being validated by someone with no agenda. It felt good, and I felt seen.

The therapy was working for me but the antidepressants were not. I was agitated and aggressive, and I hated that feeling, and I was only experiencing the side-effects, which was a common trait with me, having not been able to take the birth control pill for similar reasons when I was younger. Basically, prescriptive drugs just did not work with my biology. I ditched them and relied heavily on therapy and staying off the wagon. I went cold turkey: no smoking, no booze.

My thirtieth birthday approached, and as I am not one for being the centre of attention, yet feeling the pressure to celebrate this milestone, I held a party up north for all my family and a few friends. I was sober for the first time around my family and had no crutch to prop me up. Although I had only known

Daniel for a few weeks, he was my touchstone, and we agreed that whenever I got overwhelmed we could just go out of the room and take a break.

I was utterly in love with Daniel's family. I adopted them as my own, as I did with all my friends' and boyfriends' parents in my life, searching for that family embrace wherever I could find it. They were generous and kind, and it felt good to be part of a culture where family and family loyalty were sacrosanct.

I was working a lot and Daniel was filming in different locations around the world, so I went with him to some of his jobs, hanging out in his trailer without any pressure on me, and I liked it. However, my job was just causing permanent pain; attention from the press was still high. After three months together, while we were on holiday in Sorrento on the Amalfi coast, Daniel asked me to marry him. He proposed one evening in the grounds of the hotel down on the balcony terrace overlooking the Tyrrhenian Sea.

Daniel told me later that he had been trying to ask me for days, but his plans kept falling apart. Trying to find the perfect moment kept being scuppered – one night I refused to go for a walk because I had overeaten and had tummy ache, on another night we drove out further up the coastline and found a restaurant with a fantastic view, but a woman with a yapping dog turned up. After a beautiful dinner Daniel ordered another plate of spaghetti vongole, which I thought was odd, and still the dog continued to yap as the sun went down and the view disappeared. Finally, with a full belly to prolong the moment, his second attempt was dashed.

I loved Daniel, and I heard myself say yes to his proposal. We were not living together at that point, and just before we met I had been advised to buy a flat and get on the property ladder. I found a one-bedroom flat in Holland Park, which fell through. Now we were engaged, Daniel asked me to move into his newly bought flat, which was on the outskirts of London. I did not want to move that far out, though; for me, leaving central London was not yet on the cards. It had taken me years to establish a home properly in London, and someone asking me to leave was a wrench. I guess that's when I started to die a little. I was abandoning myself and my needs altogether for his. When we went to buy an engagement ring, I bought my own, and when he expressed a wish to also have one, I bought that too.

The press was still writing me off, and though the good-time girl and maneater headlines had gone, no one ever positively commented on my work, and the permanent bullying from journalists was affecting my mental health. I was always doing my research, always rocked up to work fully prepared. I knew my interview style was good. I knew I asked interesting questions and had an inquisitive mind, but still I hadn't developed any confidence in it or, more worryingly, in myself.

Like any self-employed business, the industry was very up and down. I was going through a dry spell, and after being careless with my finances I was forced to take out a loan to pay a tax bill. After all these years I still hadn't learned how to manage my money. I just could not understand it. Work opportunities were diminishing, but that had happened before, and I was sure it would turn around as it always had. I have always been given opportunities, and things always appeared when I needed them, despite how choosy I was.

We started making wedding plans and putting together a guest list; it was the first and only sign I needed to decide not to go down the traditional route. I suggested to Daniel that I'd like to go away to get married and not do all the seating plans and invites. I could not give a fuck about a big wedding. It was about us alone, and I did not need the stress and aggravation. I was pleasantly surprised and over the moon when he agreed. We told our families, and everyone was totally fine with it.

I organised my dress and shoes, and Daniel got together an outfit for himself. I had the something old, borrowed and blue stuff sorted and the rings had been bought. We decided on The Cotton House on Mustique, where we could get married in a Catholic ceremony in the little church just off the runway. The hotel manager was our witness, and it was as simple as that. All we had to do was get there, fly to St Vincent a few days later, get the licence from a lawyer, fly back to Mustique to marry, then get on with the honeymoon. It cost me, but it was worth it for the privacy.

The night before the wedding, Daniel and I argued about old shit, my past being a constant source of quarrels, and despite it being the eve of our marriage, it happened. We slept apart in the traditional style that night, and I lay there exhausted. Were we really doing this? Were we ready? I kept asking myself what more I could do that I hadn't already done to get him to trust me.

The following day I prepared for my big day alone. I blew-dry my hair, put on some minimal make-up, threw on the dress and got a golf buggy down to the church. The service was intimate, beautiful and emotional, and I felt a lot of love between us.

The wedding photographer took pictures during the cere-mony and a few outside the church, but I declined when he suggested going around the island to take more wedding pictures – having been photographed relentlessly for the past thirteen years, it was not how I wanted to spend my wedding day. Instead, we had a lobster lunch, I changed into my white embroidered bikini, and we sunbathed and picked shells. It was a lovely day. I was relaxed and in my happy place, on a beach under the sun.

Keeping it from everyone and out of the press had been achieved, but as we were leaving, a newspaper called to speak to the hotel manager about whether we were there, finally sniffing us out, but we were going that day, and he didn't tell them anything. We'd done it; we'd married in privacy.

In the early months of my marriage, Amanda, my agent, decided to cut ties with the agency we were at and go it alone, and I opted to go with her. She was the closest person to me; I trusted her, she knew everything about me, and I felt confident we could achieve great things together. We began to get meetings and to cultivate my next phase, but with all my financial troubles I needed to get some work fast. Daniel was getting roles here and there, but we needed something more consistent and permanent.

Despite all our worries, we wanted to try for a baby and I thought because I was thirty we should get going. I had never been pregnant before, so I wasn't sure how fertile I was. This thing could take months. But to our surprise it took three weeks. I rang Amanda to tell her the news, apologising for being pregnant and the impact it would have on my career and, subsequently, hers. She laughed at me. 'Melanie, are you joking? This is wonderful news. Congratulations! Do not worry about work; it means nothing.' She assured me that I would be fine, that we would work with it, around it, whatever it took.

The speed at which this all happened did not feel odd to me, and even though some saw our relationship as a whirlwind, I did not. We met, were engaged, married and pregnant in nine months, but it was what it was; it was our path, not to be measured by others. Judgements made about your life are endemic when you're famous, but I tried to not give a flying fuck what people thought. Hurt seeped in occasionally, and anger burned at the injustice, but focusing on the fact that jealousy was always at its core helped alleviate some of the pain.

Being pregnant was interesting, to say the least, and I hated it. I hated the sickness all day and felt my body had been sabotaged. It made my skin crawl, every nerve ending was on the outside, and people associating my current state with me and Daniel having sex mortified me. I experienced horrifying nightmares throughout the pregnancy where I did not bond with my baby. I woke up in cold sweats, crying, but relieved to find it was a dream. Despite having a rough experience throughout the pregnancy, though, I ultimately looked forward to having my baby.

I was photographed everywhere. I was hassled by men in cars on my trips to do pregnancy yoga, and the paparazzi did not leave me alone. It made me feel exposed and depressed. I did some work during this period, doing a few bits and bobs for Carlton Television, and Amanda was getting me some good meetings, but compared to the 90s I was not doing much. Times were changing and the industry and I were going through a transition period. Peaks and troughs were ever-present in my sprawling career, and in the trough was definitely where I was professionally at this time. But I was keeping busy preparing for the baby, knitting clothes and trying to stay well mentally and physically. Daniel wasn't particularly attentive during this period, and would oscillate from being supportive to trying to exert some control. It was confusing. I had to escape to Amanda's a couple of times throughout the pregnancy to get some peace as our arguments continued.

Despite all the yoga and breathing exercises I had learned, my baby was not showing any signs of arrival, overshooting his due date by a week. I was at total capacity and completely swollen from my face to my feet; a blimp and seriously overweight. I was admitted to the Portland Hospital so the doctor could take a look at me. He decided I should be induced and get this labour going, which I agreed to. We were there for hours and nothing happened, so he gave me another dose of something. We stayed overnight, and by the next day, still nothing. Since I still had officially another week before the danger zone, I asked to be released to go home, and the doctor agreed.

I tried very painful acupuncture to get my labour going and was eating a super-hot chicken jalfrezi every night; anything I could do to try to get my body into delivery mode, but it was not meant to be. One week later, I was back in the hospital and being induced one last time. The paediatrician assured me this would be like horsepower, yet still, nothing happened. Not one single contraction. It was decided I had to have a C-section.

I lost a lot of blood but we both made it through. He looked like an overcooked chicken, the poor boy. He had been in there way too long. My connection with this little man in my arms made me so happy, and despite the nightmares I suffered, the love flooded in. As I breastfed, nurtured and cared for him, my newborn baby, Roman, filled a gaping hole in my heart, and for that I was truly grateful.

Chapter 9

After the operation, the lower half of my body felt utterly disconnected from my top half, and I was all over the place. Just because C-sections are seen as a routine operation does not mean they are not also massive things to recover from – seven layers are cut through. It is not nothing, and boy did I feel it. The nurses pushed me to get up and get at it, which I know they have to do, but going to the loo for the first time made me petrified and nauseous, thinking if I pushed too hard I would split myself open and lose half my insides to the basin below me. So visceral were my fears.

The saving grace of the horror was my deepening connection to my son. I also enjoyed the embrace of my hospital suite, relishing being held by the system. It was rare for me to be looked after. I was nervous about going home and I did not want to leave.

As advised by Amanda, I announced the birth in the papers. At first I was irritated at the suggestion. I could not understand why I had to. I wasn't royalty, and it wasn't anybody's business, but my agent said I should, so I did. I took the advice and assumed she knew best.

After five days I was discharged, and like most new mothers I had a plan I would stick to, but it all went out of the window pretty rapidly. I was breastfeeding on demand and sleeping when I could. Daniel and I took it in turns to care for him, but of course the nights were mine to conquer. When Daniel got a job, Roman was only four weeks old. It was a small part in the new Lara Croft film, *Tomb Raider*. He left for Greece to film with Angelina Jolie, who is, in my opinion, the most beautiful woman in the world. I was postpartum and felt unattractive, undesirable and fat. I was a slave to feeding, my sense of self was gone, and I was insecure about him going. It was Angelina, for heaven's sake, and I could legitimately feel jealous for the first time in my life, couldn't I? I didn't share this with him, but I felt abandoned and bereft. I put a brave face on it and buried my fears, not wanting to show any weakness. We needed the work and some money coming in – God knows it was all going out. We were in serious debt and we needed a miracle, and deep down in my gut I had faith that one would be delivered.

Six weeks into motherhood, Amanda called me with a massive opportunity that had come in. Mark Wells, the head of Carlton TV, was casting for a daily chat show with Des O'Connor for ITV. They were looking for a female co-anchor, and wondered if I would be interested. It was a great opening for me, and the possibility of working with such a big name felt a little unreal.

As a child, my parents hadn't watched Des's chat show religiously, but I did know who he was and I had seen him on the *Morecambe & Wise Show* many times. He was an all-round entertainer with a wealth of charm and impeccable comedy timing, who always delivered with a massive smile, and I was looking forward to meeting him. The date was set for the following week; however, I was amongst a list of ten other TV presenters, so I was not going to get my hopes up. I decided to just go with the flow and see what happened.

Roman was permanently attached to my breasts, and I hadn't had a proper adult conversation in months. I had to find a route back to the Melanie Sykes they were probably hoping to meet, the one I, too, had been missing. I was still in maternity clothes and lost in action.

The day of the casting arrived, and I pulled an outfit together and got myself looking good enough for a meeting. Daniel drove us into town. I fed Roman in the car before I went in so as not to lactate during my slot. I hadn't left his side since he was born, so I didn't know how long I could go before I started leaking. Then, with breast pads in place and praying they would hold out, I went up.

I was charmed by Des from the get-go; he was a warm-hearted, friendly person. He made me feel at ease and told me we had something in common – it was the Boddingtons advert. After I had done the unexpected second ad, the ad agency ditched the spoof format and went into a concept with an animated cow called Graham. Des reminded me that Graham appeared in the latest advert on a cartoon version of *The Des O'Connor Show*. I had seen it in passing but, not really being a watcher of telly, I hadn't taken it in. Nuts.

We chatted and talked about Roman and my work as an interviewer. It was fun; I felt it had gone very well and my breast pads had held out. I got in the car, fed Roman, who was grizzly without me, and we drove home. A few days later, Amanda rang to say I was down to the last two women and had to do a chemistry/screen test with Des.

Daniel and I were super excited. It felt right, and if all went well I would finally have some regular work. We could get out of our financial hell and start breathing properly; we just had one more mountain to climb.

This new show was being modelled on an American hit programme called *Live with Regis and Kelly*. I was sent some tapes and studied them. They were loose in style, relaxed and having fun with celebrity guests, and they drank from mugs, which nobody did on British TV – these things were always props not to be used or only in the ad break. They were much more natural than anything else that was on our daytime schedule. The older man and younger woman dynamic was fresh on TV. The age difference wasn't apparent to me as I don't see people in those terms, and I loved being with someone who had a lot of experience. I found safety in that. I felt looked after.

We were given some subjects to discuss, and I was told to bring some ideas to the test. I decided to wear lower heels, mindful of towering over Des, and not wanting them to have any reason not to choose me.

I was so nervous and tripped down a few steps on the way into the studio. 'Falling for me already,' Des laughed. Always cheeky and full of fun. The test went well after that, and I was pleased. When I got home, I knew if I didn't land the role there was absolutely nothing I could've done any better. As with the Boddingtons advert before, I was satisfied with what I had done, but I desperately wanted the gig. So as the clock ticked on the decision, I prayed.

The day had arrived where I would find out their choice. I asked Daniel if we could get out of the house and just go for a walk. I couldn't stand around waiting for the phone to ring. While strolling round the duck pond at the local park, I got the answer. Amanda called and said, 'It's yours! You got it.' I laughed and cried and felt so grateful. Amanda told me the show would be called *Today with Des and Mel* and how incredible it was that my name was in the title. I didn't question that they had shortened my name, even though I never refer to myself as Mel. I was overwhelmed by everything and did not want to rock the boat, so I said nothing. It was such a coup.

First, we had to record a pilot, and if that worked the show would be commissioned off the back of it. If all went well, we would start filming in September, just one month away. Daniel and I were exulting at the news as Roman gurgled in his pram, utterly oblivious to this momentous time in our lives.

The pilot was shot 'as live', which meant recording it without stopping, in a perpetual flow, as if it was going out live to the nation. The subject matter for the top of the show was settled, and the three guests were booked. The style for the clothing on the show was discussed, and the team were toying with either a classic daytime look or a bit smarter. I was into my overdraft facility at the bank, so Amanda lent me some money to go shopping. I bought new black trousers and a dark blue silk blouse from an Italian designer; it was smart and more appropriate for the evening, but I felt good in it and insisted that I wore this over my more casual choice. I wanted to look good; I wanted to feel good. I was still breastfeeding; my body wasn't back. The design of the trousers made me feel slimmer, and I felt the best I could possibly with my baby weight, and the top hid any signs of my maternity bra and ever-present breast pads.

The wardrobe department agreed to this more chic look, so they matched Des's outfit and tie to mine. The show's style was set – a bit of primetime in daytime, as it was described, and that is how we did it. The pilot felt fantastic, and the way it was set up helped me with my previous sensitivities around filming. We had the autocue to get us into and out of ad breaks, which meant no remembering lines. I did not have to wear an earpiece because Des was hard of hearing in one ear and his other had to be clear for listening to guests, and there wasn't any point in me having one if he couldn't hear any direction from the producers. I was free. Instead we got all our cues from the studio floor written on boards and were given hand-signal countdowns. It was liberating and much more comfortable for me. It was incredible that with just a few tweaks of the mechanics I could actually focus on doing my job, and not have to endure it – all thanks to Des's needs. It had never occurred to me that I could have asked for help with all my limitations, I thought I just had to suck it up and deal with it as had happened before.

The pilot was received exceptionally well at the network, so we were commissioned for three months to see how we fared.

The show was an overnight success. However, I was mortified the day after our début because the *Sun* had nothing to say about the show's content, only highlighting that the shape of my nipples had been visible through my top. With a huge picture to prove it. I was very embarrassed in the production meeting the following morning, as it was all men around the table. This was the biggest paper in the country, and this is what they resorted to talking about. I asked the wardrobe to get me a more padded bra so it wouldn't happen again.

Production meetings were fun, but I was never confident

enough to vocalise any ideas I had in front of everybody. I knew it was best for me to just bring it fresh to the live shows. The work behind the scenes was intense to make the show look as good as it did, and the whole team worked round the clock.

Even so, it was gruelling for me, leaving my newborn baby, travelling from the edge of north London all the way down to the studios in Teddington, south London. It took me an hour and a half to get to work every day, on a good day, then it was another hour and a half back – if I was lucky. I was on the edge of my seat all the way home, desperate to get back and see my boy and try to unravel all that had become knotted within me for good or for bad during the long demanding days. The schedule was that we did a live show on Monday and then two shows on Tuesday – one that went out live and one that was pre-recorded for Wednesday. We would then have a day off, before returning on Thursday to film another two shows – one live and one pre-recorded – which would give us Friday off. It was doable, but the two-show days were brutal.

The schedule was relentless, and I didn't know how I was doing it. I was getting thinner and thinner and living on my last nerve. There was so much work to do that I had hired a nanny, but she couldn't help me at night. Roman was now one and had still not slept through the night. He was always awake and wanting our attention. He never settled down alone and was only happy when sleeping with us. Finally, after a year of broken sleep, I had to be radical and contact a baby sleep expert. 'Controlled crying' was a thing at that time – when you left your child for intervals to cry until they got themself to sleep. We gave it a go – it took three nights, and then it was done. It was hard for us all.

There was a permanent tension between Daniel and myself, too. He would ask me about flirting with guests. I was already self-editing on the show to try not to be over-friendly with anyone; I felt under surveillance. I was tired after work and I didn't want to come home to these conversations. I wanted to relax, not speak, just unwind and hold my baby.

The show received a nomination for the best daytime show through the Royal Television Society, and on the night of the event we were not allowed to have a plus one, so Daniel stayed at home. I was on pins because I knew Daniel was in a mood about it, but there was nothing I could do. It was just the critical production team, me and Des.

When we won, it was so bloody exciting, but afterwards when we were having our photos taken I kept being touched up by a TV personality, who would not leave me alone. He was grabbing my breasts and being a complete pest. I felt sick. I told Des, and he was fuming and asked if there was anything I wanted him to do. I said no because I didn't want to make a fuss. My big night was tainted by this, and I couldn't go home and confide in Daniel because I felt he would blame me. I couldn't come home and celebrate either, as Daniel was asleep and I didn't want to rub his nose in my success because his career wasn't thriving as he would have liked. I was constantly playing down my wins and unable to share my angst when things weren't working out.

At the weekends, when we went out as a family, people were constantly staring at us and crashing into our personal space, peering at my son in his buggy. The constant attention was unbearable. I've always struggled with the fame bit. Many people I worked with felt like they didn't exist without their fame, but the loss of my anonymity was the most significant loss of my life, and I spent years mourning it. For me, my job was a job, not an exercise in vanity or even a vocation. This job saw me imprisoned under a microscope, hurting me badly and inevitably impacting my life.

But I did enjoy talking to the guests who came on, especially those who were a massive part of my childhood: Lenny Henry, Bruce Forsyth, Noel Edmonds, beloved *Coronation Street* stars and people in the business for smiles, who were on programmes that were not based on judgement and ridicule, the polar opposite of much of our current TV climate. I was over the moon to meet them all – so many faces, three guests a day, five times a week. It was never a dull moment and mostly such a hoot when we were actually on air. The live show was the most present I felt at any time, because everything else had to fall away for an hour and I was hyper-focused on the job at hand and able to enjoy it. I was always prepared and had done the homework, so I could let go a little. I trusted Des implicitly, he had my back and I had his. Much was made of our chemistry and avuncular relationship, and that 'chemistry' grew into mutual love over the years.

I observed and learned a lot about showbiz people and their bullshit while doing *Today with Des and Mel*; most guests were charming, some were sneery and demanding, while some totally believed their own hype and, on occasion, were rude to me. But we were flying high in the ratings. The show was a smash hit with every age group.

I started being offered Saturday night entertainment shows, 'shiny floor' shows, as they are called in the business. The first was *The Vault*, which was a complicated game show that was part pre-recorded and part live. Davina McCall had hosted the first season but she had turned down the second because she was too busy, so I was asked, would I be interested? Everyone said these offers were golden opportunities and it would be dangerous to turn them down. They were somehow perceived as a gift, and I was advised that it would be unwise to not please the management. It felt like I was dealing with the mafia and I had to say yes.

I did a run-through of *The Vault*, which is where you go to a hall or a room somewhere and enact the mechanics of the game with potential contributors and game-show people to test the format, with me as host. I got the job. The money was good, but the stress levels were higher than anything I had experienced. These were big Saturday night shows, which were of paramount importance to the channel for revenue. Massive advertising deals are secured on the back of this type of format and the bankability of the host. I hated the responsibility of holding an entire show myself. It just wasn't for me. I didn't enjoy it. I felt sick all week in the run-up to it, then was high on adrenaline afterwards – although that wouldn't last very long before the dread for the next week would kick in. It was a rollercoaster. I was permanently tearful and disconnected, and I found I could not enjoy my boy even on my days off because I constantly had to do my homework for the upcoming shows.

The top of the show for *The Vault* was always traumatic, as I had to deliver a lengthy monologue on autocue explaining the complicated rules; I had to walk and talk, down some stairs, around the set and finally end up centre stage. Tempo, punctuation, clarity, warmth, energy and marks had to be hit, and one particular day it felt like none of those things would come together. Panic rose, and mid-read I lost it and began to cry. I was led off the stage, gasping for air. A nurse was called, and she took me into one of the side rooms off the studio floor, which was usually earmarked for guests and contributors. The nurse was kind; she opened her kit bag and handed me a paper bag. I was surprised when she asked me to breathe into it. It worked. I was staggered at how simple the tool was to regulate me.

She was gentle and helped me find my breath. When I was calmer, she asked, 'What do you need, darling?'

'I need to see my son,' I said simply.

Roman was just one, still a little baby, yet only three months after he was born I had started this show and worked nearly every day. As a result, I was carrying a complex cocktail of high-level anxiety mixed with managing other people's expectations of me, all while carrying an abundance of mother's guilt and loss. It was too much.

Daniel brought Roman to the studio, and it helped to hold, see and touch him. His presence brought me to my true purpose. It was what I needed. I felt valuable, worthy and connected, and I felt like something – a person with a heart to share – which was received and visibly appreciated. My tiny boy calmed my fraught energy and cooled my fired nerves. Until it was time for 'action' once again.

The show did, however, give me one hell of a career moment. Every week we had £100,000 to give to someone in the studio or home. When the money wasn't won, it rolled over to the following week. The channel wanted it to keep rolling over, but as the host and as, I think, like a viewer, I thought it more fun to see people winning a six-figure sum every week. That made more sense to me. The production team knew the contestants well and knew their strengths and weaknesses in terms of their knowledge, so they could screw them on the big money questions if they chose to. It was my first season and the sixth week of a rollover. The money was now £700,000, and Mary, a student from Liverpool, was so close to the win. Three subjects to choose from, one killer question, and it was all hers.

'For 700,000 pounds, what does an arctophile collect?' I asked. I was willing her on when she announced 'teddy bears' with her beautiful scouse accent. 'Correct,' I screamed, and shot up into the air to celebrate – I nearly hit the roof. Anybody would have thought I had won it, the way I reacted. I jumped up and gave her the biggest hug. She had shafted the system, and I, for one, was elated.

On my days off from the show, I shot magazine covers and spreads and was interviewed for countless magazines. But, unfortunately, more of my words were being twisted into headlines skewed to suit the salacious thirst of the tabloids. At home, the nanny was holding the fort, sharing a diary of Roman's activities and any happenings I missed, and I was leaving her notes of things I thought needed doing. I had a brilliant cleaner, Ligita, who I barely saw, but I knew she was keeping an eye on things.

I landed advertising campaigns, and everyone pushed me to take everything on offer. I had no time to sit back and listen to my instinct. Instead, I was shoved around, told where to be, how to be, and what to be. With zero fight, I succumbed and conformed. I was the thinnest I'd ever been, and when I see photographs from that time I can see a woman so stretched emotionally, a shadow of myself, a shell that breaks my heart.

Daniel was in charge of the money. I rarely looked at it; I was too busy making it and was trusting that he was on top of things. When we moved into a bigger house, our outgoings skyrocketed and spending was getting silly. Yeah, the bank account was healthier, but I wasn't. I was just not happy at home. I was missing my boy and it tore me apart every day.

These were the days before social media; as far as I was concerned, people loved *Des and Mel*, but I'm sure not everybody did – we just never heard about it. We were gloriously ignorant of any hate. Needless to say, it was a blissful bubble until I heard of a stalker. The channel received threatening letters against me; they must have been worried because a police escort was arranged to get me safely to and from my car after the shows. I didn't ask any questions; I didn't want to know.

I was pregnant again, planned but, as before, we conceived very quickly, and as we entered our third season of *Des and Mel* I announced the news live on air to surprise Des and our audience.

I was in Des's company more than I was my own family, which created a closeness between us but also friction, sometimes. I was hormonal and overworked, and he was getting more stubborn and controlling around the show, having a tight grip on production, and it was intense. The producers would often ask me to back their ideas because, bless Des, he did not like saying no to me. A producer even hid behind my wardrobe door one day in case Des came to knock, not wanting him to know he was in my room talking. The truth is we were both tired. There was a lot of pressure on us, and Des, now in his seventies, was expecting his fifth child.

I was frustrated and, to be honest, angry. I didn't want to be the breadwinner, I wanted to be at home, but I simply had no choice. A lot of money was being spent, but Daniel was being very picky about the offers coming in to him, while encouraging me to keep going.

I was heavily pregnant on the second season of *The Vault* and, due to the timing of the birth, would not be able to do the last three shows of the run. The channel had already secured Gabby Logan to replace me, but she could not do all of them, so they asked if I could please hold on for one more show, which I did not want to do. I was hugely uncomfortable and not fit to do it. The adrenaline that coursed through my body during these shows wasn't good for me, let alone the baby, but I felt powerless and not supported in saying no. Yet again I was advised to keep the channel sweet and do as they asked.

When *The Vault* was nominated for best game show the following year, I was told by Mark Wells via my agent that if it won I would not be going up for the gong, but Gabby would instead. But I was not to worry, as *Des and Mel* were up for the best daytime, so I should be grateful. I was fuming. She had only covered a few shows in my two-season run. I was flabbergasted. 'But why?' I asked. The answer was because the rollover had got to a million pounds and had been won live on air on a show she had hosted, and because it was a record figure, given away on an ITV show, they wanted to use that clip, so I was to remain seated. I was livid. That night Gabby was sitting with Mark in front of me, and I was flanked by Des and Daniel. I waited for Gabby to say something about how maybe I should go up with her if we won. Neither she nor Mark said anything. When the announcement and clips were shown, Davina McCall swung round and looked at me like, what the fuck?! The cameras were everywhere, so I couldn't react. We didn't win, though, and I was glad.

Something in my mind was clearly switched on that night. Never again would I feel beholden to these jokers, but I also felt trapped.

Just six months ago I had given birth to my beautiful new son, Valentino. I was overjoyed to have another boy but the birth had been extremely traumatic – I'd lost a lot of blood and we had both been in danger. The frightening experience left me with post-traumatic stress, and I'd only spent just under three months with him before I had to go back to work. I was back in therapy when the awards 'do' happened. I was not in a good way and I was totally over the whole media circus.

My marriage was miserable, too, which added to my grief. I was always where I didn't want to be, nobody was coming to save me, and my morale was really low.

The truth is I was downright depressed. I was snappy and angry and absolutely hated my life. I was trying cognitive behavioural therapy with my therapist, who also suggested that Daniel and I have couples therapy, but it wasn't beneficial. One day my therapist had to change where he could see me from our usual central London address to The Priory, a famous establishment for helping people with mental health conditions and often addictions. Unbeknownst to me, I was followed from my home by a paparazzi guy, and the papers rang my PR agent to ask why I was at The Priory. I couldn't believe it. So I had to tell the papers that I was having therapy for post-traumatic stress from my birth, which had a total of fuck all to do with them or anyone else for that matter. The threat was that they would have insinuated that I was in treatment for drug and alcohol abuse if I didn't comment.

When you're doing daytime and primetime shows, you're supposed to be a model citizen and free from scandal. Anything could be deemed scandalous, the way things were written up; normal human behaviour was considered dangerous to your persona. It's not like now when a person's wellbeing is considered. You did not matter. You were a commodity for all. Back then, you were a puppet and you did what you were told. I had a regime at work and at home.

During this time, we were doing renovation work on the house, which was costing us a fortune, having a boiler replaced and a general beautification of the place. One day we arrived home and when I put the key in the lock and heard 'rain' I was momentarily confused because it was a dry day. Then I realised the sound was coming from inside the house. It was literally pouring in the living room. The boiler had broken, and all of our beautiful renovation work was ruined. The wallpaper, the fabrics, the new furniture, the fixtures and all the fittings were destroyed. We did get it all back on insurance, but still, that house was over, so we moved into rented accommodation in Hampstead. We got the repair work done but we never moved back in. It was a relief for me to be back in central London, where I did not feel so cut off, and where we were close to the children's schools, which was much more convenient. It made me feel a little more human again.

Then, after a successful run of shows, *Des and Mel* was not recommissioned. It was the end of an era. Mostly I felt sad and anxious about the future of my career, and then I felt relieved. I was back at home, and that's when I realised things were not as they seemed with Valentino.

Chapter 10

For the first time since the children were born, I was now fully rooted at home and more present for them. But that came at a price – I was worrying about the dramatic reduction in our family income. We hadn't saved any money while I'd been working, so there was a constant thrum of anxiety about our financial stability and future.

Being at home, though, meant I could observe my family better; the boys were no longer with a nanny, and I could see their dynamics and what was happening with them more closely. Our gorgeous Roman was a whirlwind and always so chatty, his little voice filling the air and always seeking our attention. Valentino was the complete opposite, and it was a tricky balance to find in parenting. When I brought Valentino home the first time, Roman asked if we could put him in the flowerbed, not wanting him to live in the house. I struggled to divide my attention between them and I felt that I'd failed to blend them, as Roman continued to be a little dismissive of Valentino.

Mine and Daniels's relationship was also a challenge. I was drowning in the relationship and had lost myself completely. I had changed my personality, how I dressed, and how I communicated with people. Daniel trusted no one, so to keep him happy I felt I couldn't be too friendly with anyone and couldn't talk about our dynamic to anyone either. I too grew to trust no one, which cut me off from the outside world.

I was fully embedded in my family's dynamic when I was told that my nana was in the hospital and I should get home as quickly as possible. So Daniel held the fort at home, while I travelled north to see her. Grandad was already in the hospital when Nana was admitted, so the family had to go from ward to ward to visit them both. It was a crazy situation. When I arrived, Nana was sitting up and chatting. I sat on the bed with her, and she gave me the download on the other patients and the nurses. She was in a mischievous mood and surprisingly perky. The following morning, mum got a call saying Nana wasn't very good and that we should all go there. So we all came and sat around her bed, talking and taking turns to sit nearest her and also visiting Grandad, who they had moved to be nearby. We had been there for hours and at lunchtime ordered some sandwiches. When they arrived we all started to talk about them, whose was whose, and handing them round, and then we noticed Nana's breathing change and slowly, slowly she took her last breath. I watched intently how quiet it was and felt blessed that it had been like that for her. I had never seen someone die before; this was my favourite person on Earth and I had watched her pass. I could only feel great blessings for being there. She is missed, but not completely, because I feel her presence every day.

I had to get back home to my family – and find work. But still I was watching the boys and picking up on their signals and behaviour. Roman was curious about everything, strong-willed, but not disobedient, and always on the go; Valentino had always been more mellow, much quieter, and a more placid child. He did everything on the doctors' targets for his age – growth was 'normal', he moved onto solids at the usual time, walked at the appropriate times, and started saying a few words (the first being 'strawberry') in the 'standard' time frame. But Valentino didn't engage in the usual way. I tried to play tea party scenarios with plastic food, a teapot and teddy bear guests, but he hated it. Instead, he would put his foot through it. He was fixated on fabrics, he loved to touch and play with the labels on everything, could fully engage with wooden Thomas the Tank Engine train sets and was fascinated with the underbelly of the mechanics – he didn't use any of his toys conventionally.

Valentino was such a beautiful child and he loved to be cuddled and held. He let us know precisely how he felt when I did not want to be somewhere and was very sensitive to noise and smells. For instance, he hated going to the indoor play centres, with the oppressive atmospheres and layers of sounds of kids enjoying themselves. It was hell for him, and he would scream to leave. Juggling both children and their needs and preferences was difficult. I had never used dummies with the children because I wondered why I would stop their only way of communicating. It didn't make sense to me. During mealtimes, Valentino always looked like he was daydreaming, just staring out of the window. He became picky with food, but I kept putting these things down to him just being him, being a different personality to Roman, and not thinking that there was anything else going on.

It was around this time that we had to get Valentino inoculated. We decided to do separate jabs because it was when there was a bit of noise about autism and the MMR jab in the press, with claims that the booster could cause autism – although this theory was later discarded as untrue. Tino's first jab was for protection against measles, and he became exceptionally poorly afterwards. He had terrible cold-like symptoms for two weeks straight and he stopped speaking entirely. The smattering of words that he had been saying were all gone. He was distant and checked out more often, and when we said his name he did not turn to face us. He wasn't pointing at anything either. Daniel was away on a trip when I noticed that Valentino was withdrawing further – I could not ignore it any more, so I decided to take Valentino to our doctor.

The doctor told me that, from what I described, Valentino might have 'glue ear', which could be treated with grommets, a tiny tube inserted into the eardrum to allow air to enter the middle ear and clear the blockage, or, in fact, he might be deaf. It was a worry, and the test was difficult as he wriggled relentlessly and did not want to be there. But it was evident during the process that hearing was not his problem, so we were referred to a top paediatrician at the Cromwell Hospital. Daniel came home.

After a series of investigations we were told that Valentino was probably autistic. I did not understand what it meant, and the description we were given was unclear, but it was delivered in a way that we should see this diagnosis as a problem. I was confused and frightened of the unknown. My only reference to autism was the *Rain Man* film, where Dustin Hoffman played Raymond Babbitt, a savant with an extraordinary ability with numbers. I have never been somebody that searches online to investigate medical stuff, and I was not going to start now. I prefer to rely on clinical experts. Needless to say, Daniel and I were concerned and we were dealing with the diagnosis in completely different ways. I wanted to stay positive for Valentino, but it felt like hell, and I had nobody to talk to. To reveal my fears to Daniel felt dangerous, and I didn't want to be dragged down by his feelings. What I needed was positivity and to be lifted up. Unfortunately, we were just not there for each other.

Tino's behaviour was challenging for us to manage; he had 'meltdowns' everywhere we went, even trying to climb out of his car seat on motorways. He would scream everywhere we went, if he couldn't cope with the atmosphere. He hated having his haircut, the sight and sound of scissors around his ears and head would cause him significant distress, and he felt like a ticking bomb in every place and situation. People would look on with disapproval; they were extra curious because they would recognise me and they looked on with their judgemental eyes and intrusive stares.

Over the months of wanting to escape this living hell we were in, I tried to adopt a positive and cheerful attitude, but it felt impossible to sustain. I did not feel equipped for the challenge of looking after both children, all whilst trying to resurrect my career into something more meaningful, but not wanting to go headlong into the crazy pressures of what had gone before. In my time out I had decided I was no longer going to be a shiny floor show presenter and instead I wanted to do some meaningful documentaries, more cerebral things, which were more in line with my interests – art, travel, film and books – and I also had an idea for a comedy drama.

For now, though, the focus was all on Valentino. We took all professional advice that was on offer and agreed to more tests on our son. We were told we should explore if his autism was behavioural or in his DNA, so he had blood tests, and one appointment had Tino's head covered in electrodes to measure brain function. He just ripped them off his head in indignant rage. In the end, I, too, called time on all these investigations and decided to pull the plug. I realised I didn't need to know 'how' he was autistic, medically or otherwise, just that he was, and I desperately wanted to focus on how to help him with the overwhelm he was feeling everywhere we went. Even while these tests were going on to establish where his autism came from, at no point did anyone investigate if either Daniel or I were autistic ourselves.

We were finally put in front of a brilliant paediatrician who simply said if I had a child diagnosed autistic I should go and see Dr Stella Acquarone, who had a private clinic in Hampstead. Stella believed in early intervention to help children suffering from overwhelm and was very much into connecting parents with their children using therapeutic means. She offered a three-week course on communicating with your child and helping the child feel grounded. It was all based on therapy – play therapy, couples therapy and family therapy.

It was expensive, but it had to be done. We went into debt to pay for it, but I felt I had no choice. We were at a loss and this seemed like the lifeline we needed. My instincts were screaming at me to go for it. Daniel was a bit more sceptical, more guarded and more suspicious, and he found it challenging, as did I. The therapists focused on the dynamic of our marriage and zoned in on our relationship with each of the children and any home atmosphere that might be compounding problems. It was an invasion of our private life, which I relished, needing the backup that I hadn't found anywhere else. The only person who knew how unhappy my marriage had been was my agent. It was a relief to let people know professionally, and as it was shrouded and wrapped up in helping Valentino I felt sure that Daniel would not back out. I was willing to do anything to help our son, and I was happy to be able to discuss my marriage in a safe space that Daniel could not wriggle out of. It shone a light on our parenting skills and where we were not doing so well, which felt humiliating and shameful. It wasn't what Daniel wanted, but he stuck it out for the sake of our son. The best thing was that Valentino was beginning to talk more and more and express his needs in a way that he hadn't before. The therapy was working and was worth its weight in gold.

It became clear that all this time we had been trying to fit a square peg – our gorgeous boy – into a round hole – the system – and it was not going to wash. So we just stopped trying. We put an end to all the standard kids' stuff and started to tap into his desires, not ours. We got back to basics; we reconnected with nature, and got rid of the mountains of plastic toys we had that would overwhelm any child. Letting that all go was profound for me; I had to get to Tino's level to see where he was and go from there.

During therapy, I had the disturbing realisation that I'd always made myself available for Roman so he didn't feel neglected with me having a second child. I was fighting against the feelings that I had felt throughout childhood, but in doing that I had overlooked Valentino. It was harsh and it hurt, and I tried not to beat myself up about it – which was not easy. Roman, who hadn't been enamoured with me bringing this imposter home, had still not bonded with Valentino and was eager for my attention. So Valentino, my quieter, more under-demanding child, had been left to sit on my hip and listen, and there wasn't any space for him to engage.

Autistic people are super sensitive, and the vibes in our house were not good. My autistic boy would not be inclined to fight against the constant surge of demands, conflict and palpable unhappiness in our home. It was just too much. Daniel and I were forced to share our marital differences in couples therapy. The specialists talked a lot about boundaries, which helped me realise how enmeshed I was with Daniel, and I had to face the harsh reality that I had demonstrated no self-will for six years. Nothing for me, not even time.

I moved into the spare room and started experiencing life a little bit more on my personal terms. This included going to bed early to read, listening to music I liked and having space to process and think without behaving the way I had previously always fitted into Daniel's schedule. It was a game changer, and I emerged like the children, starting to tap into my own needs. With the support of the therapists, I gained the courage to demonstrate boundaries and know that I was allowed them. It felt good to have people care about my wellbeing.

I was getting back to myself and getting healthier for the kids. In the course of this, I learned to get to Tino's level and build from it. I was able to create things he liked to do, play with trains and fabric, which he loved, and we started to talk; I would give him language and narrate our play, and he began to come out of himself. Every word he had heard over his three short years was present and they started to pour out of him. We also learned to let Valentino know what we were doing and give him the heads up when doing anything out of the ordinary so he wouldn't be surprised. So, for example, when we went on holiday we showed him pictures of the hotels, the caravan, the plane, the trains or whatever it was. All these pre-warnings reduced the overwhelm and fear, and it worked.

The course ended and we were left to get on with our lives. There was a moment mid-course where our whole way of living had been broken into pieces, and I wondered if we would ever be able to lasso it all back together. But here we were, more settled, trying to rebuild in a new way, and it felt good. We weren't left completely stranded after therapy, though, as we visited the clinic weekly for much-needed aftercare while we oriented ourselves back into everyday life.

A few months later, Valentino became a source of concern again when his health turned for the worse unexpectedly. We noticed his face was swollen and he did not look right. We called a doctor, who thought it sounded like an allergic reaction to something, so he prescribed an antihistamine. Over a few days, I could see the drugs were not having an effect, and he was ballooning around his middle too. I took him to our GP, who did a protein test on his urine; the results we were told were dangerously high and indicated something was wrong with his kidneys. We took him yet again to the Cromwell Hospital, where we were admitted as a matter of urgency.

We were told that he had nephrotic syndrome, which causes the kidneys to leak large amounts of protein into the urine, and can lead to swelling of the body and tissues and more significant problems of catching infections. It affects around one in every 50,000 children a year; our little boy was one of them.

'How dangerous is it?' I asked the specialist, and without an ounce of delicacy he said, 'If he doesn't respond to steroid treatment in the next three days, it could cause a fatality.'

I was devastated; my every nerve ending was on fire, but I emotionally armoured up and set foot into the fray.

It took three adults to pin down Valentino to get the cannula in. I was destroyed watching him fight and helping them hold him down, feeling his body resist like hell to get us off him, but it had to be done, and the course of steroids began. He tried to rip the cannula out of his little wrist and hated the taste of the bitter pink medicine; trying to get him to swallow meant we had to hold his nose so he would open his mouth. He hated the treatment, but we kept pinning him down to administer it. It felt barbaric but necessary.

I slept by his bed and did not leave his side. Not leaving the hospital even for a minute to get air. Daniel came daily and brought Roman occasionally to see his brother, not wanting to disturb his schooling any further.

After three days, Valentino still hadn't responded to the medication. Protein was still spiking in his urine, and I was praying, praying, holding him, playing with him and praying some more. The doctor's words were a permanent fear in my head. Three days. Finally, on the fourth day, the protein had reduced, and his swelling had started to subside. I was told that these episodes of this syndrome could last until he was seven or eight. The truth is it lasted into his early teens; he had many relapses over the years, which was always a worry. Checking his urine regularly and subsequent intermittent steroid consumption was the advice we were given to keep him alive. It was hardcore, and a constant concern. The steroid treatment affected Tino's mood, which was difficult anyway with his existing sensitivities. It was hard to know what behaviour was him and what behaviour was from the side-effects of the steroids. Still, they were keeping him alive, and that was all that mattered. How much this little boy had been through was insane. He was only three years old at the time.

With some of the questions about Valentino now answered, we found a home to move into. We sold our home and moved to the suburbs of Hampstead; it was lovely, semi-detached with a garden, three bedrooms and one bathroom; it was beautiful and it had a great vibe.

We moved in, but still the marital boundaries were in place.

I started to resurrect my career again in a different way. I finally said goodbye to Amanda in an agent capacity, and our friendship also ended, which was sad after all these years. The reason why I made this split was because I wanted to tap into my creativity. After being a prolific reader and diarist for so long, I thought it was time that I enrolled on a writing course, and I started to write a comedy-drama with Simon Golding.

Simon had come into my life after he had seen an interview where I'd said *Kes* was my favourite film of all time. He had written a book about making that film, and we bonded over our love of the film director Ken Loach. Our comedy-drama concept was taken from my experience of behind-the-scenes of *Des and Mel*. The BBC read our script and was interested in it, but they wanted to buy the concept and elbow me out of the writing and the production. I was disheartened and declined. I was looking forward to being involved in casting; even Des was interested in playing a version of himself after I sent him the script. I would have been happy to advise and be behind the scenes. I had read countless scripts, running lines and making performance notes over the course of my career and relationships. Such is my love of film that I have always fancied myself as a casting director, or director instinctively understanding talent and knowing how to nurture it.

I was determined to never do any big game shows again and only co-present in future, because I liked the safety of this structure. I wanted to flex my intellect once and for all, too; I really wanted to work for Radio 2 – my dream station, which I had been itching to be on for as long as I could remember. I'd done some commercial radio, but it had felt like a glorified sales job, and I realised it was not for me. I just wanted to talk and I hated all the incessant reading of competitions and sponsored content. Radio 2 is where I thought I belonged, but it was off limits for the time being because I was told the head of the station was not a fan of mine and I could never get a meeting with them anyway.

I was still in therapy, and my therapist encouraged me to unlock my creativity and independence in all areas of my life. I joined a gym, and enjoyed it. I loved how it made me feel and how I could transform my body. Things were opening up but my marriage was shutting down, and after one too many battles I finally called time on it. I could not do this in front of the boys any more, and I asked Daniel to leave.

Chapter 11

The separation was actually a relief, and it had been a long time coming. In my mind, now it was done, I could start living again instead of existing.

The truth is that Daniel and I are chalk and cheese. I am, and have always been, free-spirited. My life was not meant to be lived in a cage. I am an eternal optimist, and I trust and love people with all my heart. I don't want to ration that. Daniel is the complete opposite. It was a shame because it overshadowed the fun he was capable of having and how entertaining he could be. Our arguments were never loud, crashing events, but the vibes were evident, and the kids must have felt everything too. It didn't matter how many years we had together and how involved we got; I felt he didn't believe in us. There was nothing I could do to change it. In turn, I was programmed, maybe from my Catholic upbringing, to feel that marriage was for life, so it felt somehow wrong to end it. But my spirit was wasting away, and I could not be there for my children if I continued in this vein. Despite all that, I had to mourn the loss of our relationship.

People commiserated with me, making massive assumptions about the situation. A reaction that I thought was weird. It was my choice. I didn't feel like I was a failure; I had tried and it did not work. Instead, I congratulated myself for braving divorce – which is enormous – and going it alone and saving my sanity and peace so I could be a better mother to my boys.

My therapy was going well, liberating me, and it was a fantastic outlet for sharing all my problems in my new life and exploring why I had always been drawn to conditional love. It was a lifelong pattern. You are not lovable if you are not doing as you are told, was my unconscious limiting belief.

I could now focus on sorting out my finances; not supporting another adult was a relief. I sold the cars we had, getting back to what I wanted to drive and taking care of only me and the kids. I was putting myself first, as the clinic and my therapist had taught me. Women are programmed to serve everyone else without any sense of self, which is dangerous and unhealthy. It's a very convenient narrative set by men. Women are considered selfish if they put themselves front and centre, but by doing that my life became calmer and more manageable. I could be me without any boundaries; I could breathe.

The boys were tiny, and they saw their father often. The first weekend the kids had to go with Daniel was extremely hard. After closing the door on them with a weak and fake smile, I slid down the wall, sat on the floor and sobbed, staying there for a few hours. I let go of all the tears I had not cried and mentally wrestled with myself, but my gut was right: this was for the best. Eventually, I peeled myself off the floor, pottered around the house, put the radio on, cleaned my make-up brushes, did some bits and pieces on the vegetable patch I had started and ventured back into the kitchen to try my hand at cooking again.

I was on a reboot after spending time prioritising Valentino and his health. I told people in my personal life about Valentino being autistic, but I hadn't announced it publicly; it was a family matter and I wanted it to remain private for now while we were getting our heads around it. I would share the information when the time was right.

I also had to keep a focus on earning money, so I found another agent who I hoped would get me into Radio 2. The former head had resigned after the Russell Brand and Jonathan Ross incident, and Lewis Carnie had landed the top job at the station, and he liked me. So I was finally in at Radio 2, where I could talk without interruptions, have fun, engage with guests and be myself.

Luckily for me, my first pairing on a show was with Aled Jones. We had a good rapport, even though – and not to diminish our chemistry in any way – I do get on with most people. You have to be a complete twat for me not to be able to find common ground with you or like you, although that did happen several times with various future pairings. Aled had a free and easy style, he is generous, funny, and a brilliant broadcaster. I adore him. It was the first show I was assigned to do for the station, and I ended up being there more on than off for the next fifteen years.

I was still doing some TV on the side – really just to pay the bills, because my hatred of cameras was still a hindrance, I still could not be my best in front of them and be my authentic self. I was a completely different person away from the cameras, and it felt like I was living a double life.

I was doing some filming for *The One Show*, which felt like starting over. I was filming a few videos for them, agreeing to appearances where I wasn't presenting, as I was advised that being seen on certain shows would remind people I was still around. When the co-host job became available, I was asked to audition for it. It was awful. I could not use the earpiece, I had no idea how to do gear changes on subjects, and, deep down, I did not want to get back into a daily situation and never be around for the children when they got back from school. The production team asked me to come in and have another go, but I declined. It was not the gig for me.

I also auditioned to present the *Strictly Come Dancing* spinoff show *It Takes Two*, and I failed that audition miserably. I could not do fast-paced shows and, again, listening to cues and countdowns in my ear while engaging with guests was impossible for me. It was sensory overload, and I could not master it. Of course, in hindsight all this connected with my autistic sensitivities, but I had no understanding of this at that point.

I did stand in for Paul O'Grady a bit, who had a hugely successful five o'clock slot on ITV. His producer, Bert, who produced the first three years of *Des and Mel*, had another hit on his hands with the incredibly gifted Paul. Paul O'Grady was an understudy for Des a few times during our run, which were some of his first appearances on daytime television as himself, not Lily Savage. He had been considered quite a risky character historically, due to the character of Lily Savage: irreverent, saucy and more suited to primetime than daytime television. However, he was now showing what he was about for real, and I thought he was the bee's knees. I still do.

Paul had the odd day off from his show, so I was pulled in to cover for him at the last minute. I was well versed in live TV, and the good news was that I did not have to wear my earpiece and got all the cues from the floor, and the format was simple. I wasn't very good at all the pantomime and stage stuff, which I found excruciating, but the chat bits I settled into and felt okay. I did a few more of these last-minute appearances to cover for Paul, and they were as enjoyable as they could get with all my sensitivities, but I knew it wasn't where I wanted to be.

Things were going well, and I signed with Morrisons to be a new face of the brand, which I continued with for a few years. I loved shooting the commercials and working with directors, so these fun days brought some much-needed moments of joy while I was going through my divorce. Making some money was a relief and Ligita, who had now morphed into my right-hand woman and closest confidante, was always with me to make the juggle easier, consistently by my side in support.

While work was going well, personally things were not so great. The divorce was getting messy. Daniel's lawyers were coercing him to ask for what they thought he was entitled to, which was to live in the way that he had been accustomed to, and were suggesting I pay him maintenance. The whole thing was fraught, unnecessary and painful. We ended up having to go to court. Luckily the judge threw out Daniel's lawyers' claims. What a colossal waste of money and time, both things that should have been spent on the children.

I decided to leave my marital home, rent it out, and move the kids back where we could walk to school and feel less cut off. It was a rental flat that I could have the option to buy, which I thought might be possible, but when I finally decided to sell our suburbs house I lost a lot of money on it, and sadly I didn't get around to buying again. We were living hand to mouth for a while, and I chose to travel with the boys and have some experiences over buying more bricks and mortar that didn't exactly work out for us the last time. I was concerned about putting a big chunk into something and then struggling to afford to live day to day. It was a gamble, and doing things like that was not my forte. I was going through an expensive divorce, and it was horrendous. I was trying to juggle a lot and still focus on getting work.

I wanted to do what *I* wanted to do after seven years of living in a way that wasn't me, dressing in a way that didn't reflect me. I was rediscovering who I was. I had a specific look for *Des and Mel* and all the sexiness had been robbed from me. I started to buy myself new underwear and new clothes. I was in shape and felt like a woman again. Then I began to see a new person.

I had reconnected with a guy who had worked on *Des and Mel*. James was working on the Paul O'Grady show; he'd started out as a runner on *Des and Mel* back in the day and was now a director-producer and Paul's right-hand man. I'd always liked him. He was down to earth, a Northerner like me, and pretty chilled. We ended up hanging out at an industry party, getting drunk, and snogging. It was fun but felt weird to suddenly be with someone new after all these years. I was footloose and fancy-free, and I could do as I pleased, but it felt odd and something to get used to.

Soon, it was in the papers with all the 'mystery man' bollocks, a total yawn fest. We had fun, and he was on a level with me. He knew the business well; he understood its demands. Eventually, we moved in together. He helped me open up and explore my creativity, encouraging me to start drawing and painting. This was when I realised I was pretty good at composition, and I enjoyed these discoveries. I was unearthing the creative child in me, and I was surprised by my natural talent. I was dabbling in watercolour without any technique and drawing everything. His family were wonderful and creative, and I felt I was getting back to elements of my youth and who I actually was. The TV industry had thrown me about, and my marriage had morphed me into something else, something that just wasn't me. A strange version of myself that I had to take on to survive.

James helped to open me up again and live with fewer restrictions. We talked about having another child but when I spoke to an obstetrician they said at my age of thirty-eight I would be described as a 'geriatric mother', making the idea seem less appealing. My drinking was revving up again, though I didn't focus on it and didn't share this with my therapist. My old demon had come back to haunt me. James and I started to argue all the time and eventually, after just over a year together, we called time on the relationship. It was fraught and just not working, and I was not happy. He was a good guy. We just didn't work out romantically. But we are still friends.

My fortieth birthday was coming up, and I decided to go to La Colombe d'Or hotel in Saint-Paul-de-Vence, a beautiful place in the South of France where the food was world-renowned. I booked for five days, and a friend was joining me for a few of them. I spent the time sketching, reading, eating, drinking and smoking while mourning the breakdown of yet another relationship. Unfortunately, when my friend came out, she got sick and spent her time in our darkened room for two days, which was a disappointment; however, I did have a dinner arranged with Richard and Judy and their children, Chloe and Jack, to celebrate my birthday. They were great company, Richard and Judy finishing each other's sentences with the best stories. It was hilarious fun. A memory I will always cherish.

On the day of my fortieth birthday, I had to fly home ready for my radio show with Alan Carr the following day. He had a Saturday night show called *Going out with Alan Carr*, and I was asked to cover his co-host for two weeks, who was going on holiday. After I signed up, I was told that she had rung and asked if they would cancel me, as now she could do the dates. The producers told her to go on holiday and come back as planned, and, apparently, she resigned. They accepted her resignation and so my first ever show ended up being an audition. Alan's agent rang me after the show and said the position was mine if I wanted it full-time, and I said yes. The regular work was terrific, being with Alan, who I loved, and on the station I wanted to be on. I felt happy and totally blessed. I could bring myself to it and laugh with the audience and my co-host.

My personal life was picking up, too. I was now a permanent feature at the gym. I was making new friends, using a PT called Alex – a brilliant woman in training to be an airline pilot who I totally vibed with. I was eating well, my body was changing, and I felt confident. At this point my divorce finally came through, and the day it appeared in the paper I received yet another misogynistic swipe based on one of the terms of our divorce, which was about our financial situation. The tabloids said, '*Let's hope Melanie Sykes' new boyfriend has got lots of money.*'

It would have been laughable had it not been so hurtful and unjust. I had never lived off anyone my whole life – everything I had, I'd earned through hard work and sacrifice. I had put a roof over our heads, food in our bellies, and I had been the bread-winner, so to be written off in such a way and dismissed made me seethe. A woman turning forty and independent of any man was not being championed. I tried to rise above it and find a way to not let it take me down. But privately, the injustice killed me. Still, I was pretending nothing bothered me and I kept going. When the divorce was final, I was sad, but Daniel and I were trying to find a way to be friends, and despite the headlines we checked in on each other to see if we were both okay.

The boys were getting older now, and Daniel and I decided it might be time to tell everyone that Valentino was autistic. It was the right time for us. I thought it also might help some people, including me. I did not have any friends in the autistic community, and it opened me up to hopefully making some connections and talking to mums whose children were further down the line than me. It felt good to get it out there, especially as Valentino was doing well. I did some TV shows about autism and my experience at the clinic, and people were contacting me online and sharing their stories too. It felt good to be helping and making connections. I then met my first friend who had an autistic son too. Vikki was brilliant fun, and we could share our issues unguarded and be mutually supportive. She became vital to me.

They were nine and seven when the boys really discovered each other, and they began to find each other very amusing and became great playmates. I loved to watch them laugh together, they were so sweet and oh so playful. My boys were full of fun, raucous and amazing. When I wasn't travelling alone, I took them on holiday and braved long flights and lovely new coun-tries to show them a bit of the world. I changed their names to double-barrelled names, to include mine, so there was no confusion about us having a different name while travelling.

People's reactions to me being alone with my children were interesting. Once, when I was in St Lucia having a beautiful candlelit dinner with my sons, enjoying the tropical breeze and view, the waitress approached the table and said, 'Oh, what a shame. Is your husband too busy to come away with you?' I was in shock. 'No,' I said, 'I don't have a husband. I chose to bring my children on holiday.' I could not believe, one, that she would say it in front of the children, and two, she would make such a massive assumption about our situation. I found it utterly bizarre, but this happened in some capacity every time we travelled.

Back home, Hampstead was becoming tricky for me because of the paparazzis' permanent presence. There are quite a few well-known people in the area and around it, so we were some of many who were photographed every day, often on the school run. This went on for six years or more, and hugely impacted my children and me. It was brutal and unnatural, and all I wanted to do was tell them to fuck off, but with the kids in direct earshot I had to keep calm and reassure them they were safe. Protecting children from photographers is something a mother should not have to do. They were shameless, with no regard for the mental health of my children or me.

The children and I were forced to relocate again because my flat was being sold by the landlord, but despite the issues of the area, I chose not to move far as the children were still in school, so proximity was the better option. We moved on the same street, literally one minute down the road. It was a smaller flat, but it was what I could afford, and I liked our road, so I didn't want to go too far. Ligita and I are highly skilled at moving quickly and did it using my little Fiat 500 with the roof down, shuttling back and forth. There is nothing she has not seen or heard, she is my great friend and the most incredible presence in all our lives. The boys adore her, and so do I. I do not know how I would have got through everything without her.

In addition to the presence of the paps, Hampstead was ripe with gossip, which is one element of living there that I'd never been comfortable with. I've never talked about other people's personal lives and judged them, it's not my style, but I myself had become fodder for those conversations. I was also managing unwanted attention from other quarters, and so were the boys. Roman told me that two different male teachers at his school were asking him questions about me and mentioning me all the time. No child wants to talk about their mum at school, and I was livid. I warned both of the teachers – one by phone and one in person – that if they did not back off I would go above them to speak to the headmaster and create a formal complaint. Needless to say, my chat with both sorted the bullshit out and stopped it from happening. Men were saying whatever they wanted to me out on the street, too, in front of my sons, and I was just holding it together, not reacting so that my sons weren't affected. Between that and the paps, Roman just stopped walking with me, instead choosing to walk ahead, breaking my heart.

It was around this time that I heard about a social media platform called Twitter. I was not remotely interested in sites like this – hell, I didn't get an iPhone until an agent encouraged me to get one so I could receive emails at any time, which sounded abhorrent to me, but I indulged him anyway. I was on location in Scotland when my makeup artist encouraged me to set up an account and showed me how to use it.

I surprised myself and really loved it. It was so much fun — apart from the trolling. I could be chatty and silly; I made sexy jokes and was being myself. I soon had about 3,000 followers, and it was good fun. I was making friends, even meeting up and going on nights out with a gang of girls who all seemed to gel, and it was fun and games. I did not take Twitter too seriously; it wasn't at that time anywhere near as toxic a place as it is now. I ran some commentary during Premier League matches, as I was obsessed with football, watched all the games, and knew everything that was happening. I was also cheeky, playful and totally me. I think I shocked people because, as far as they were concerned, I was Mel from *Des and Mel*, and some people had me cast as a perfect princess, which I've never been. Some people even thought my account was fake because they did not associate my humour with the person they perceived me to be from the telly, which I found amusing.

I landed a new lunchtime show on ITV working with Gino D'Acampo, called *Let's do Lunch*, so we met and then got started on it. Over the next few years, that show was an endurance test for a variety of reasons. I never complained, as I didn't want to lose my job. I had mouths to feed and rent to pay.

All in all, I was, by my standards, happyish, but I wasn't healthy and was getting blind drunk a few times a week, hanging out with people who were not necessarily good for me, but I couldn't see it.

My brief relationship with the trainer at the gym ended when he called time on it. I was finding it easier to bounce back from disappointment now, and took the rare opportunity to rebuild in private. I also decided to take a ten-day trip to Seychelles to regroup and heal my wounds, and I returned a new woman. I had also found myself a new agent.

Melanie Cantor was, at first, my friend. We met when we were cast as judges for a talent contest to find a presenter on GMTV. She had been a successful TV agent for many years and then retired. I was moaning one day about work, and she suggested that maybe she could come out of retirement and help me along. I thought it a fab idea, so she did, and she was brilliant. She was strong, knew me well and cared for and supported me. It was the first time I had felt looked after and cared for since Amanda, and it felt good.

Together we landed a new gameshow pilot called *My Man Can*, with Mark Wright. It was for ITV and in a large Saturday night format. The primary role was the female one for a change, and it was big and fun and following an existing successful German format. The concept was that women gambled on the success of their husbands in various tasks in a roulette-type scenario, with chips and a green baize and me as a sort of croupier. I met Mark, who I loved, and we started doing many run-throughs.

It was a fun time in my professional life, but my personal life was about to go through a rollercoaster of change, thanks to some interaction on social media with a guy who was playful, persistent and intriguing. I was in such a good place it felt like fun, and I just didn't see the drama coming that would unfold.

Chapter 12

I had become amused by a guy flirting with me on Twitter. He was funny and different and didn't say the obvious things to me. He tried to get my number through all the people I was talking to, but without success. I was happily single and wasn't looking for a relationship at all, but after a few months of him trying to get me to follow him so he could speak to me privately, one morning I just felt like it, so I did. The DMs began, leading him to get me to download WhatsApp to continue the conversation. He was cute, funny, physically my type and confident. He also had a child, which I thought was good – going out with younger people, I always felt the issue of children would be problematic down the line.

Jack and I had chemistry from the get-go and he was fun and carefree. We were messaging regularly, and we both decided it was time we should meet in the flesh. This was before the explosion of online dating, so it seemed risky, although nobody bats an eyelid now. Everyone is a stranger until you know them, and people meet random people daily in all sorts of scenarios, but because I met him through social media our relationship was later deemed reckless by the British press.

I spoke to a few of my friends about whether I should meet up with him or not. The general consensus was why not, and that's what I felt too. So I agreed to go on a date with him. I joked with a friend that I would send a 'code red' text if I was in danger. We were joking, though, and I was sure everything would be all right.

I waited at the bar and ordered a drink. In previous chats he told me he was a trader of some description and was thirty-one and 6 foot 1. As he tapped me on the shoulder, I realised the latter two claims were a lie; he was much younger and much shorter and was late because he had driven up from Dorset, which was a bit odd because he had also told me he lived in London.

I didn't say hello. Instead, the first thing out of my mouth was, 'You are not thirty-one.' Jack just laughed. 'Seriously, how old are you?' I continued. 'I've just turned twenty-five,' he said, 'and if I had told you my age you would not have met me.' He smiled, and he was right, and I liked it.

His chutzpah and charm won me over. I couldn't give a crap about his height, age or what he did anyway. He told me he was a lead roofer living back with his parents. None of it mattered to me, and we had a perfect time. We had such fun drinking, being raucous and having crazy chemistry. After that, it was a done deal. Jack ended up becoming my boyfriend.

Within a week I travelled to Dorset to meet his family and son. I fell in love with all his family. They were just a dream. He opened me up and encouraged me to be playful and take risks. I'd been thoroughly indoctrinated into being a famous person, always looking over my shoulder, so I threw caution to the wind and went with my feelings for Jack. He was also brilliant with my son Valentino, particularly, and helped me organise my finances better. In addition, he was so helpful, showered me with silly romantic gestures and provided me with fun. Our families blended well together, and I was happy.

One night, I was home and he was in Dorset when he messaged me to say, 'I've left a message on Twitter for you. You have to respond.' The tweet read, 'Hanging out the back of Melanie Sykes'. I was really shocked and didn't know how to respond. Not wanting to seem prudish to him, I pretended it was funny. I asked him to help me come up with something instead of telling him to delete it. I just wanted to be playful with him. So he told me to put: 'Well, put your phone down and get on with it.' We both thought it funny, but although I didn't really want to post it I had so few followers, and it was a joke, so I ignored my instincts. Neither of us could have predicted what a shit storm we had just ignited.

The next day my agent called me and said the press had read it and were printing all of our messages from Instagram to date. I found it crazy that our silly conversations on the platform were monitored. It didn't occur to me that journalists would follow me and that there was a kind of surveillance in play. I only had 3,000 followers at that time, so hardly anybody knew about it until the exchanges were all sensationalised and taken out of context, then they were put out as fodder to millions of people as the tabloids cashed in on me once again. It went from being seen by my tiny community on Twitter to splashed all over the papers. Shared with millions of people. I was mortified.

When we were flirting online it had been just fun, but out of context it was made to look scandalous. The press said the messages were disgusting, and I was shameful. I was embarrassed and worried that the boys would have to deal with it at school, as all the kids' parents were talking about it. I was braving the school run, being photographed while doing it, and could feel the judgement from the other mums. It was a joke.

I was summoned to ITV to apologise to the boss and explain myself. I was fuming all the way up to his office in the lift, flanked by my agent and PR agent. 'This is ridiculous. I don't want to do it. Why do I have to apologise to this guy?' I said. My PR agent kept saying, 'Just do it, say sorry, and it's done.' What a fucking joke. What has this newspaper story got to do with my ability to present shows? Surely the public wouldn't turn off my shows because of it?

My PR agent was in overdrive. As advised, I had to do an extensive interview and photo shoot with a Sunday magazine to further explain myself and clean up my reputation. It was all so toe-curlingly embarrassing, and what a bizarre industry. A total circus that exploits the person in the limelight and where financial gains are had by all bar the person at the centre of it. It is sickening and wrong.

When the journalist asked me about the text, she had understood that we were having sex when the messages were sent. I could not believe it. 'When was the last time you were having sex with your husband and on the phone at the same time?' I asked. She seemed flustered and did not respond.

The climate was that the press was obsessed with my relationship. They just did not leave us alone, they were everywhere, all the time. I was in love and happy, but the constant pressure on us was draining. In addition, information was being unearthed about Jack, and concerns I had were starting to set in. It turned out that he had been messaging other famous women but I was the only one who had taken the bait.

Jack brought up marriage, and I told him from the get-go that I was not interested; I had not long divorced. For me, marriage had been reduced to the merging of assets and then the separation of assets. There was no romance in it, and I was happy doing what we were doing. It was not for me. He had no interest in having another child, so I thought that was that. But he did persist with the marriage question.

In the months following, I felt he became erratic and impulsive. Jack was chain-smoking, drinking and consuming an unhealthy amount of Red Bull; he was ramped up. I began to recognise the signs of jealousy in our relationship.

Work was going well for me, and *Let's Do Lunch* was a hit, and there were some amazing people on the team, especially our director, Dave Skinner, who I'm friends with to this day, but I was enduring a lot of crap and unprofessionalism, and I was also juggling everything as always. And there was still the show with Mark Wright. We had shot the pilot in Germany on the actual set they used for the original show, even using the German crew. With the run-throughs being weeks before and my memory as it was, I suddenly realised I needed a crash course on the game's dynamics before we shot the pilot, so I got the series producer to go through it with me, and it all came back to me. The pilot was a success, and the show got commissioned.

I was starting to change my image slightly, too, as my agent Melanie Cantor had recommended I use Gary Cockerill, a makeup artist whose style was uber glam, with big hair and lashings of makeup. I had to steer him not to overdo it, but sometimes he could not help himself. It was a very sexy look. Gary first styled me for the National Television Awards, and as always I doubted my looks, never feeling truly beautiful and forcing myself to brave the overwhelm of the red-carpet gaze and demands to smile. The bank of flashing cameras caused heightened anxiety and a permanent ache. Other people seemed to enjoy it, but I was merely enduring it.

Once inside the event, the pressure to mingle was on. I was trying dry January but I hadn't made the whole month, and I decided to have a drink to calm my nerves from the red carpet, and then to drink some more to feel comfortable in the room. The next day the head of entertainment at ITV, called my agent and warned me not to drink too much at these events. I was devastated, and it pissed me off because Holly and Phil were the presenters of the channel's most valuable daytime TV show and they were being celebrated for their drinking and colossal hang-overs on air. I, on the other hand, was only drinking in front of purely industry people, and she felt the need to pick up on and remark on my behaviour and flex her power. Her reputation did precede her; I had heard that she could be hardball, particularly with women, and now I was experiencing it first hand. When I went to Germany to film the pilot for *My Man Can,* she flew out to oversee proceedings, and because she was there I was the only one who didn't celebrate the record's success, instead choosing to go to bed early, avoiding her judgement. The rest of the team all partied until the early morning hours. It felt highly unfair; I was a forty-two-year-old woman being treated like a child.

This wasn't the only flak I was getting at work; I was being ridiculed and pushed around and disrespected quite a lot in various parts of my working life and so I started to explore different requests that were coming up. My radio show with Alan was a welcome break from all these shenanigans; it was good to have a weekly broadcast where I could represent myself away from the constant derogatory narrative about me, away from the pressures, and just have fun with him and our loyal and brilliant audience.

Alan was doing a New Year's Eve TV special, and his agent, the late Adisson Creswell, had asked me to go on. Adisson was the most significant agent for comedians in the country at that time, having broken the ceiling of where acts could perform with Lee Evans at the O2 Arena in 2007. He was a character himself, and I liked him. We had been having lunch and hanging out professionally, and he wanted me to explore stand-up myself. He found me funny, and I thought the idea was interesting, so we were percolating the idea of my 'learning' stand-up for a documentary, for which I started to write lots of material.

The New Year's Eve show was to be pre-recorded, and would have lots of famous guests just being silly as well as some live acts. I did not want to go on the show; with all the press I had had recently and the shaming that had gone on, I did not want to risk appearing on anything that might see me be degraded or diminished. Addison assured me that would not happen and that he would protect me.

However, that night I was disrespected by a colleague, and at one point, when I was recording a 'piece to camera', I looked down and he was lying on the floor just staring up my skirt, which he thought was funny. I was horrified and screamed. He got up and I threw a drink all over him. It was all caught on camera. I watched the show on New Year's Eve to see how that moment had been handled and was horrified to see that they had edited it in such a way that they did not use the footage of him, only footage of me losing it. And they had taken the moment into a 'break bumper', a trailer that gets people to come back to the show after the break and not switch channels. There was no context to it; I just looked crazy and had been thrown under the bus once again. After that, I never spoke to Adisson again. I was so angry, and not long after, he died. I have always felt sad that I hadn't resolved my upset with him.

I was drinking increasingly in private and being very cagey about being out and about in public. I knew I was drinking too much, but it was difficult because Jack and I were taking it in turns, him wanting to slow down one minute and me the next; we never wanted to do it simultaneously. He was now living with my boys and me, and we had become a blended family. Everything we did was photographed, though; the paps lurked at the bottom of the street and would photograph me kissing him goodbye when he went off to work. They would describe the pictures online as a PDA, a 'public display of affection', but the only public around to see it were the photographers stealing images of us for their own financial gain. Jack was slagged off for not being good enough for me, and I was slated and questioned because he wasn't famous and what was I doing with a lead roofer? It was warped and damaging for both of us, but we had to try to shake it off and focus on our families and work.

We went to Dorset weekly and hoped our boys would bond. We rented a little flat next door to Jack's mum and dad so we didn't always have to descend on them every weekend. I loved the lifestyle, and Dorset was so beautiful, a great escape from London. It was a slice of nature that was lacking in my life, and we were so close to the sea. We explored the Jurassic coast with our children, which was so much fun.

I was feeling that this could really work between us, despite the glaring warning signs. All this time, Jack never gave up on wanting to get married; he talked to me about it a lot. He is very persuasive. The truth is I changed my mind because I loved him, I felt like everyone deserves a wedding, and just because he was younger than me I didn't want to deny him the opportunity. It wasn't because I wanted the whole marriage story. I know the press like to write me up as someone that believes in a happily ever after and fairy tales, and pursues that narrative, but in reality it has never been me and as silly as it may sound I purely agreed with it as a gift for him. So I finally said yes.

Jack's family were so happy and excited for us, but I hadn't spoken to my family for quite some time. Between divorcing Daniel and where I was at this point, communication with my family had diminished. We all went on holiday together, but I didn't feel part of the family. I was there with the boys, who were still so small, but there was a disconnection that was painful. I felt like an outsider. Trips up north became non-existent, and nobody was coming down to see me either. I'm sure all the news stories made life difficult for my family, but not as much as it all hurt me. Living in survival mode was the norm for me. I rang my mum to tell her I was getting married and invited some of the family. It had been a long time, and it was an emotional call for me, as they weren't a part of my everyday existence. Mum said of course she and Dad would be there.

Jack knew of my complex relationship with my parents and the emptiness it caused, and later he would be able to use this knowledge against me. Loneliness dogged me in or out of relationships and I could never find my feet properly – it was one drama after another, and I was not equipped to deal with it. I let everyone rule me, push me around, I believed that others' opinions were more valid than mine and I was deeply unhappy but refusing to go there to that dark space. I was a walking contradiction because I was also amazingly razor-focused regarding my children, and I was high functioning in many ways. I was running a home, a career, and managing the different characters coming in and out of my life – of which there were many, both personally and professionally. My most significant and important commitment to me was raising my two boys, though.

My friend Vikki and the group of girls I met on Twitter were great fun, and we were vibing. Vikki and I were particularly close because of our sons' shared autism diagnosis, so we decided to do some fundraising for Dr Stella's clinic so that people who could not afford to pay for private treatment could get the same help for free.

Vikki came down from Scotland to brainstorm ideas. We came up with all sorts of hare-brained schemes and decided, because of my last Boddingtons advert, we should drive an ice cream van down from John O'Groats to Land's End, selling ice creams all along the way. It was perfect. First, though, we had to get the van and learn to 'pull' ice cream. I got really good at it, and it was hilarious fun. Then I had to have a refresher course on driving a manual vehicle, and Vicky had to learn to drive from scratch so she could share the driving. I was useless in the van, and after some pretty treacherous driving by me – taking bends on two wheels in a borrowed ice cream van you are in fear of tipping over is not good for the nerves – I retired and let Vicky do the rest. We laughed so much at ourselves and each other. It was daft fun. We didn't raise that much money, but we did raise awareness and made some hilarious memories to boot. We had a total riot. There are still things that happened on that trip that make me roar with laughter today at the most random times, and it was a welcome light relief from my normal life.

I was in constant therapy still with my therapist from Stella's clinic. She helped me navigate the boys' needs, my work, my new and very public engagement and the mounting issues between me and Jack. Despite mainly being hungover every time I went to see her, I hid my drinking from her. I sat clutching a Lucozade bottle like my life depended on it − it was the only thing that worked for the nausea and banging head. I never discussed my drinking with her, but I did share some concerns I was having with Jack.

It seemed that the more attention we got, the worse the relationship dynamics became. His family were a big draw to the relationship for me too, and I rationalised everything by his fantastic parents; he could not be all bad if his parents were so amazing. It wasn't possible. One Sunday, his father took me out clay pigeon shooting. It was something I always wanted to do, but I had been under the impression it was what the gentry did, not people like me, and was surprised to find out it was accessible for anyone. I realised I was left-handed but I didn't have any technique, so I listened to his instruction, and it was apparent that I was a decent shot. I became obsessed.

Despite the peace and love I found with his parents, I couldn't find it consistently with Jack. If he couldn't get hold of me he became suspicious and angry, and I could see the signs that his jealousy was a gazillion times worse than I was used to. He hated my male friends and would blame me for how he felt. I tried to be calm and not inflame situations, but I also tried to teach Jack that whatever he felt was something he needed to work on himself and that it was not something I could alter. But unfortunately he wouldn't listen. I did love him, but I found myself trapped once again. As I've learned through my relationships, the creep of toxic relationships is sometimes slow and intermingled with good times and good sex, which can cause disorientation and confusion amongst bitter arguments. It was hard to distil what was happening, even though the feelings were familiar. I couldn't join the dots.

Chapter 13

Jack had introduced me to his friends. They were all just kids, of course; they were starting out in their lives, thrill-seeking and generally doing what early twenty-somethings do. I could hang with them because I could hang with anyone, but I was not stimulated intellectually. It didn't occur to me that that was what I needed; after all, I had once had a boyfriend who thought humans had shared the Earth with dinosaurs. He had shared this information with such conviction that I nearly doubted myself. When I asked what his source of information was, he emphatically declared, '*The Flintstones!*' I could not stop laughing, even though he was far from joking.

I was not sharing my life with people on my wavelength in any way, shape or form. Instead, I was seeing the charm in it rather than the incompatibility. Me being ever the optimist, I was going with the flow, finding my own mental stimulation as always with my reading, but socially it was just drinking and being silly. I had more in-depth conversations with Jack's parents, staying up with them talking long after Jack had gone to bed. I was closer in age to them than I was to him, so it was a no-brainer that that would happen.

The trust between us had gone. He was getting nasty, saying horrible things to me. I started drinking to have the courage to verbally defend myself. So when I drank I got brave and retaliated, telling him his flaws and how he was hurting me. Over time we got further and further apart, and we started arguing more. It was confusing because our sexual attraction was fire, and all our arguments were resolved this way, never with discussion and solutions.

When things were good and if he was working on the weekend, I would go to work with him. Climbing up scaffolding to sunbathe while he worked. We were sometimes so close, like best friends, but it was punctuated with times when he was wildly jealous, and I thought he hated me.

I was still doing *Let's Do Lunch*, and Jack picked fights at the most inopportune times for me, always heavily orchestrated to cause the most effect on me. He sometimes phoned me while I was in makeup at work to continue arguments. I was in tears in the makeup chair and crying off my makeup artist Helen's good work. Finally, she had to grab the phone and tell him to leave me alone. I had a live show to do. He harboured arguments until the last second, too. Once he had been in a mood all Sunday, and I didn't know what was wrong. I had to get up crazy early the next day to go and appear on the morning TV show. I was booked to talk about autism awareness month, and just as I was about to leave, at 5.45am, he picked an argument. He had had all of Sunday to bring it up but instead had waited to pick a time that was the most challenging for me. Live TV was a struggle as it was without knowing that I would be returning to a massive row at home. Jack was also jealous of me working on filming *My Man Can*, which was exhausting, and I was drained from trying to make him feel better.

His insecurities started messing with my head and my self-confidence. I became unhappy and a little scared that I was making a mistake. I was worried that we were so deep with the wedding plans but that we might be doing the wrong thing. We couldn't afford it anyway; well, he couldn't and he'd promised me that he would pay for half of it as soon as he had the money. I used my savings for most of it and gave him more money to help with his business. We were in deep.

We were holidaying in Sicily when we were writing the invitations for the wedding. I had paid for us all to go on this trip, including Jack's son. It was our first 'family' holiday. I wanted to show my boys their country of heritage, even taking them to the town of Caltagirone, which was known for its polychromatic buildings and stunning ceramics, yet it also had a sinister vibe and was almost deserted, so we left pretty quickly. It was a bearable holiday, though, and the children were the least of my worries, as Jack was so moody. Writing the wedding invites just did not feel right; my gut told me not to do it, and even the ink in my pen was not flowing correctly. The writing was a mess, but I sent them like that anyway. The universe was giving me the signs, but I was not tuned in.

Back in London, our wedding plans were ongoing. We decided to have the wedding reception in Sherborne Abbey, which was down the road from Jack's family home. It was stunning and very grand. I was nervous about tying the knot in such majestic surroundings. I also worried about how the kids would cope with the ambience and organ music reverberating around the church's inner expansive space, so we took the children to accli-matise them and arranged to meet the vicar.

My agent, Melanie, was keeping the wolves at bay and manag-ing my work. She rang me to say that although we had recorded the entire series of *My Man Can* it would not be broadcast. The news was totally left field, and my only question was, 'Why?' She said the reason was that the gambling issue had not passed compliance and was not allowed on British TV. Although the whole premise of the show was set around gambling, the produc-tion team had spent months during filming trying to fudge this critical element and hadn't found a way to hide it within the format. It was still blatant gambling.

It was insane. We were paid in full, the channel had spent God knows how much money on its production, and now it would never see the light of day. I was surprised, as this was a new one for me. I had done plenty of pilots that did not get a commission, but not this. But I was, in truth, relieved.

Gary had been doing my hair and makeup on the show, and when I'd gone to do some dubbing and voiceover I saw myself on screen and didn't like what I saw. I looked way too glamorous and unnatural, and I hated it. So I was relieved nobody would see me like that. When the press release went out about it being cancelled, the line was that Mark and I had 'failed to understand the concept of the game'. I was fuming. Thrown under the bus yet again. This industry was a horror story.

In the meantime, we moved flats again, to the same street but a bigger place that would house us all. It was a four-bedroom with a fantastic view across London. It wasn't very modern, but the space was good. Ligita and I got busy with the move and had everything set within days. It was a significant rent increase, but Jack agreed to start contributing something, he just didn't have the money to split our outgoings down the middle. So my finances were permanently being drained.

The marriage drama increased when our church wedding plans fell through at the last minute because the local press had become aware of the arrangements, and now everyone knew the date, time and venue, and because it was a public space anyone could attend. The whole experience was going to be difficult as it was and now I was worrying about Valentino in what was threatening to be a circus. So we cancelled. I was so angry.

We decided to relocate the whole day to Sherborne Castle, to marry in the orangery and have the reception in a marquee on the grounds. It was a beautiful venue but there would be no religious ceremony, so we had to get the marriage licence and change up what we were doing. We nearly missed our appointment to get the required documentation because Jack overslept. It was such an important morning, and if we missed the window the date would have to be changed. I was so upset, I didn't even want all this anyway. I was doing it for him and he couldn't even be bothered to get his arse in gear to get out of bed. What was I doing?

When I wasn't juggling everything else, I found time to shoot clays. I was now addicted to clay pigeon shooting and was having lessons at the shooting grounds of renowned gunmaker Holland & Holland, where I was learning 'sporting'. Sporting clays is the closest thing to actual field shooting, which I had tried only once, and had killed a partridge. Someone smeared my cheeks with its blood, as is the custom marking your first 'kill', and I handed the gun back to its owner, never to repeat the experience again. It was not my scene at all. Sporting was much more my scene; in this the clay birds are launched from stand-ardised distances and angles, in layouts designed to simulate the movements of ducks, pheasants and rabbits – the latter were, for me, hardest as they bounced erratically along the forest floor. I was hitting the clays early out of the trap, not waiting for them to hover above me or wherever they were coming from. I was just quick off the mark, and my trainer thought I should have a go at the Olympic trap, which is more difficult than most other trap versions because of the distance to the targets and the speed with which they are thrown – a super-fast 63mph – and they fly out from any angle of an arc and require quick action. Jack's father, Bob, advised me to contact Peter Wilson, who had just won a gold medal competing in the double trap at the Olympics, so I did. He, too, was Dorset based, so it was easy to set up a meeting. He thought I had the potential to compete, and that excited me massively.

Peter described Olympic trap as the Formula One of shoot-ing, and I went to my first OT layout and loved it. He put me on to a coach named Martin Barker at the Nuthampstead Shooting Ground near Cambridge. I loved Martin; he was a charming, intelligent, funny outdoor man through and through and could tell the time by a quick glance at the sun; he was a total dude. He was incredibly economical with his guidance, which I liked, and big on telling stories. He was wonderful. He saw my potential and encouraged me to compete; he hooked me up with a gun sponsor, and we were getting to work. We talked about everything under the sun, even my concerns with Jack and my deep troubles. We would smoke and speak between rounds, and I loved spending time with him. It was an oasis away from everything.

Away from the shooting ground, I was in last-minute organising for the wedding, and I had done a deal with *OK! Magazine* for some pics. My friend Alan Strutt photographed us, and we gave a few approved pics to the magazine. The children were off limits, and it was just a couple of pages. The payment covered the honeymoon expense, so that was a relief, as I was using my savings to pay for the wedding and I was running low.

The day before flying off for my hen weekend, I got a call from Dad, telling me my beautiful cousin Paul had killed himself. The news was delivered in Dad's unceremonious way. I was confused; he was only thirty-one, had a little boy, and nobody knew he was in pain. Even as I write it now, it does not seem real. I loved him very much. I was grief-stricken, and my heart broke for the family. I spent the entire hen weekend drunk and had to attend Paul's funeral the following week. Everything was so surreal, and I was in deep shock. It still hurts today.

Things were rough between Jack and me, and we had a big talk about pulling the entire shebang. But finally I thought it best to plough ahead. And there was no way he was going to pull it either. Plus, I actually believed I loved him.

The day arrived, and I felt relaxed enough to sort out my receipts for my VAT returns. All my paperwork was all over Jack's mum's floor as I sat in my bathrobe, ready to post so it wouldn't be late. I had had a wobble with my matron of honour the evening before about whether or not I was doing the right thing – my mate Jo from my college days who had come over from Australia, especially for my wedding – but these pre-wedding jitters completely disappeared on the morning of the big day.

The ceremony was lovely, everything looked beautiful, and everything went well, but I couldn't brave the socialising. I struggled with mingling at the reception, always terrible with small talk, and was glued to my seat all day, not wanting to go up to the tables and talk to everyone. I also hated being the centre of attention. All the reasons I didn't want a big wedding the first time around were apparent, and I wanted to just stay back and watch everybody else instead. I blocked out the best man's speech because I knew some drivel was being spouted, so I was able to zone out, and I slowly drank. Adrenaline kept me from getting drunk, but it gave me enough courage to finally start mingling and dancing with everybody.

The day had gone well, and everyone had a good time, so I thought maybe this was meant to be. I felt utterly in love with him. The honeymoon, however, was a minefield. We both drank too much and he thought I was flirting with other holidaymakers – even my diving instructor wasn't exempt from his distrust. An argument would flare up, and I would want to talk about it and get to the bottom of it, but once Jack had me riled he would roll over to go to sleep. I was devastated. When he was happy, I was, and when he wasn't, I did everything I could to get him back onside. I felt he wanted to shame me.

We came home to start our life together, and a week later I went on a charity walk for the autism clinic. I went off to climb up Ben Nevis with Vikki, another one of our fundraisers for autism. I flew up to Scotland, leaving Jack with the boys. Vikki and I drank wine and danced in her living room until late, which was not the best preparation for a ridiculous climb, but we had fun, and I was happy. But because I hadn't looked at my phone all night, I woke up in the morning to loads of missed calls from

Jack. He was fuming and we had a massive argument. My spirit was on the floor; all before I had to do this daft big climb. Ben Nevis would be tricky, but it would be even more problematic with this extra burden.

As expected, the climb was challenging and seemed never-ending. Vikki was sick on the way up, and we needed many breaks. I talked her up that mountain. My claustrophobia was kicking in, and I had to breathe my way through it and coax her up in increments when she wanted to give up, but we eventually made it to the top. It was a glorious achievement sadly marred by my toxic husband, but by the time we hit the top I was miles away from my troubles and could be present and enjoy the moment with my friend. My only problem now was getting back down and going back to him.

Jack was working more locally than before, and I liked to say a quick hello on the sites and take him some lunch occasionally. I was doing my best to be supportive, but he couldn't handle the attention I continually got.

I wanted to go on a summer holiday, but he said he didn't want to come because he felt guilty about leaving his son, who couldn't go with us because of timing. I told Jack that if his son didn't know (he was only young and living with his mother) I didn't see what the problem was, but he refused. So after three months of marriage I still had to have holidays with my boys alone.

Jack's behaviour was getting strange, and he made the holiday hell, constantly calling and threatening to divorce me. I held it together for the boys as usual, but I was in a lot of pain.

Jack's behaviour continued to appear erratic; one day, he walked into the living room with a long straight cut on his head.

I asked what he had done and he said he'd walked into the corner of a door. He then photographed the wound and put it on Twitter, which I thought really odd.

After a huge fight, I decided to go to my friend Clare's for the weekend. I wanted to get away from him and discuss my marriage with a friend. I needed some perspective. He was vile on the phone all weekend, and I was in one big hole of a mess. He was constantly saying horrible things to me and about me whenever we tried to sort things out. I begged him to not say these deeply wounding things. I tried to explain to him that these words can never be eradicated, that they were poisoning the relationship and that he had to stop. But he blamed me and said I didn't understand how I made him feel. I was getting nowhere.

I was back and forth between my shooting lessons and doing meetings for work. The offers were coming in and I was just about to sign a massive deal for a clothing brand that my agent had been negotiating for weeks. I had a late offer to go into the jungle for *I'm a Celebrity, Get Me Out of Here*, but it was not enough money, and Jack felt unsure about it, even saying to me, 'What if you fall in love with someone in there?' I did not need the aggravation, so I declined. Then I was asked to go in to BT Sport because the boss wanted to talk to me about possibly hosting the MotoGP series. I loved bikes but didn't think I was suitable for the show. I hated live OBs (Outside Broadcasts). Whenever I had had to do them historically, for example for the Oscar coverage and any live location feed for *The Big Breakfast*, I never enjoyed them. There were too many distractions, I was reliant on the earpiece that I couldn't handle and there were a gazillion reasons why my sensitivities could not do it. I explained all this and was assured they would do anything I needed to make it work; I could hold the broadcast together and let the experts do the talking. My agent was really excited, and it was decent money and a big opportunity; I asked if I could go off and think about it, and they agreed. However, deep down, I knew they could not possibly change any of the dynamics I was worried about. With my sensitivities, I knew it was impossible for me to do live OBs.

Jack was not too enamoured with the idea of me being around all the riders either and was not best pleased with the job offer, as it meant I would also be travelling a lot. But he seemed to be holding it together and putting a brave face on it.

We got ready to go to a gun shop in central London where a drinks thing was being held, with a smattering of business conversations and some fun too. Ligita came to look after the boys, and out we went.

We met my agent and a few people at the pub nearby. I find it difficult to mix my personal life with work; I'm awful at holding social situations together and can't do introductions. If I am forced to do it, I forget everyone's names and go to pieces. The pressure is too great. I am better after a few drinks, when those fears drop away. People at the event were talking to me and not really engaging with Jack, and I needed him to be able to hold his own, but he couldn't, and he was getting more and more pissed off. Some rugby dude was loudly and unashamedly flirting with me, which didn't help the situation either. I was managing it but not encouraging it, and always worrying about how Jack was reacting. To add insult to injury, Jack was trying to give up smoking and was beyond irritable. I had not given up cigarettes with him, so after taking fag breaks outside I was having a lovely old time. Everyone was drinking, but then it was time to get home, and my agent saw us into a black cab and said goodnight.

There was tension in the cab, but I would not have a row in front of the driver, so we had to wait until we got home. I got Ligita a minicab home, then Jack and I started getting ready for bed. The boys were fast asleep. He was fuming about the night, how he hated me flirting with this person and that person. I had had enough. It was the final straw. I was not going to give him a minute more of my time, and I simply told him it was over. I couldn't take any more – he had to leave. He agreed and started to pack. He didn't have a suitcase, so he started filling bin bags, which were building up in my bedroom. He was still arguing with me, but I counted the minutes until he would be gone. I could not wait to see the back of him. He started to goad me with his shit talk and low blows, but I just kept trying to breathe and not rise to him. He was leaving; arguing for me was history.

It took all my strength not to scream, but I did not want to wake up the children. He kept saying horrible things, trying to goad me into a fight. I took my clothes off and got into bed, my heart in pieces, but I kept breathing slowly and prayed he would leave. Instead, he jumped onto the bed saying he had been talking to Daniel about me, and started throwing more accusations at me.

This was the last straw. I flew out of bed and dived into him. I wanted him out; he had been pushing me and pushing me. He wrestled me to the ground and held me down. Every time I tried to get up, he pushed me down again. I tried to scratch his face, wanting him to get off me, but he kept holding me down. Eventually I decided to let my body relax, go limp and stop fighting. At that point he got off me.

I grabbed some clothes, ran into the kitchen, found a ciga-rette, smoked it, and tried to get my head together, praying that he was packing and leaving. I was quietly crying, desperate not to disturb my children. After I smoked the cigarette, the buzzer sounded in the flat, and when I went to answer it there were two police officers at my front door.

Chapter 14

They told me my husband had reported me for an attack on him, and I had to go to the station with them. I couldn't believe it. I couldn't compute what was happening. All I had done was ask him to leave. Why did I have to go? Why could they not just assess the situation and get him to leave, as he clearly was doing? His packed bin bags were lying everywhere as evidence. Why did I have to go?

I was asking him to leave, and he wouldn't go; I had escaped a toxic marriage, and now he was accusing me of something. The police asked if I would like Jack to stay while I went to the station, which was obviously met with an emphatic no. I wanted him out. I rang Ligita to come back, but the police would not let me wait for her arrival. I needed her to take care of the boys until the morning, as it was now quite late at night. A police officer would wait with Jack until she arrived.

I woke the kids to tell them that I had to go down to the police station to sort something out; I told them Jack was leaving, and that Ligita was on her way. I promised them everything was okay and I would be back before they had to get up. They were calm and sleepy and had heard nothing. I was managing to hold my shit together; I was conditioned to handle it internally and not let loose. I had to for the children.

I was not handcuffed but I was escorted downstairs to the police car. They told me I could make a call, so I called my agent. He asked me if I wanted a lawyer and, stupidly, I refused. I needed to get back to the boys, and I thought that waiting for a lawyer would prolong the whole thing. I was also worried that the incident might get into the papers and anxious about the negative impact it would have on my ability to earn, so I did not want to make a big fuss.

At the police desk I was asked to remove my jewellery. I took my engagement ring and wedding band off and put them in a little plastic bag, marking the end of my miserable marriage. I begged the guy at the desk, 'Please do not tell the papers, as this will affect my ability to take care of my children'. He simply said, 'We don't do that,' but I knew they did. After being mugged years ago, I knew they had the option to call the press.

I had my mug shot taken and I was fingerprinted. It was an out-of-body experience, it just did not seem real. They put me in a cell to 'sober up' before interviewing me. I lay there under the blanket. There was a camera in the cell, and I felt self-conscious when I had to pee, the loo exposed in the corner of the room. I imagined the police watching me on a monitor like I was on a TV show. My spirit was crushed. I covered my head with the blanket so they could not see me and tried to rest. All that came to me was not feelings of hate and blame but the question, 'How did I get here?' It just kept circulating in my mind. I needed to get to the bottom of this, I had work to do, but I had no idea how much.

I started to get claustrophobic, and I asked the police to open my cell door a little, which they did, and then I was interviewed soon after. I tried to minimise the damage during the interview and play down the situation. The policemen asked if I wanted to press charges against Jack, and I said no. All I wanted was to go home. I told them we fought a lot and claimed the blame. I was still thinking it was my fault. I asked, 'What is the quickest way out of here?' 'Take the caution,' they replied. I didn't understand what it meant, but I did it anyway, so I signed the relevant forms so I could be released and get home to my children.

It was the early morning hours and I was terrified of getting a cab alone, so when the police offered to give me a ride home I accepted. On the journey back, they chatted about work, asking me about my co-presenters and general showbiz gossip about the famous people I knew. I was friendly, discreet and holding it together. I was going through the worst night of my life and felt I was in a vulnerable position. It seemed safer to conform and go along with their jovial vibe.

They dropped me at home in the early morning. I almost fell through the door, and Ligita was there to catch me. I managed a few hours of sleep before the boys woke up.

I knew it was only a matter of time until the press got wind of it, so I rang both schools and said there was a family bereavement and the boys would not be coming in indefinitely. Daniel was away on a trip, and I had to think fast. I called my friend Clare up north, who opened up her home to my children and me. I'll always be grateful to her for that. She organised a reliable driver to come and pick us up and take us to her. He was coming from Manchester, so we had time to pack.

Jack messaged to say he wanted to come and get the rest of his stuff, which we had now piled in the living room. I caught a glimpse of him arriving, then I turned my back and stood guarding the boys' bedroom doors. Ligita showed him his bags, and then he left. My agent came to see me to show support. He was brilliant and kind and said we would get through this. We both knew it would be everywhere. He told me that the clothing company I was about to sign with had pulled the deal, but BT Sport still wanted to go ahead. I would deal with all that later; right now I was in survival mode.

Social Services called, and I had to speak to them about the arrest and if I was fit enough to still have the children in my care. It was horrifying, but luckily I had a very understanding woman on the line, and she assured me things would be okay. Those children were my reason for being; surely they would not be taken from me? I just had to wait to see if anything would be taken further.

Halfway up the motorway, my agent called to say the story was up online; a version of what had happened was everywhere. I couldn't read it thoroughly, too frightened to see how it had been skewed. I then braved Twitter, and even with one eye closed I could see the beginnings of the abuse that I would be subjected to. The boys were in the back of the car, oblivious. I had always kept them out of any unfolding drama, and that was how it would stay. I was emotionally winded, a hole where my heart had been. One more knock and I would dissolve, but I must not fold, not now.

Clare was amazing and she got the boys sorted; she had two little boys as well, and they all just got on with being kids so I could finally let go. I surprised myself that I didn't want to hit the bottle in full. I drank a bit through the next few days but had to keep my wits about me, and my phone was blowing up. A few ex-boyfriends were calling me to see if I was okay. They had been hounded by reporters. My family and Daniel's family were doorstepped. The press were like vultures, trying to find out if I had a history of violence.

Clare and I had talked about getting some legal advice, and she introduced me to her friend's husband, a local lawyer. I wanted to see if I had a case for getting my caution revoked. The last few days had been unreal as I realised I now had a criminal record, which meant I could not travel to Australia or America, and my liberty had been affected. I hadn't realised what signing that bit of paper would do – for me, it was not an admission of guilt but simply a way to get back to my boys quickly.

My ownership of a gun licence was also potentially under threat, which cast a long shadow over my dreams of competing. There was not one area of my life that the whole incident did not affect. Jack was also calling me, begging me to sort things out with him. 'You are my wife; we have to work it out,' he insisted. But I meant what I said that night; the marriage was over. I did not want to inflame him. He had already started doing Twitter posts about the situation, which was having a ripple effect on the prolonged narrative. I just said nothing and did nothing. My PR and agent did not want me to challenge the caution; they thought it would all blow over if I did nothing, and people would just move on. But what about me? None of this was just going to 'blow over'.

Daniel finally arrived home from his trip, and Clare's husband escorted the boys by train down to him and back to school. I could now let go and start the process of rebuilding. After two weeks of being cooped up, Clare encouraged me to leave the house. All I had done up until then was pop out into her garden to smoke. I was terrified. I imagined everyone thought I was a monster because Jack was playing the victim; the press wanted me to be the villain, but he still wanted me to get back with him.

I braved leaving the house to pick up some food, and when we popped into a petrol station I saw all of the weekly magazines with my face on the covers. I saw the photos of the cut on his head from a few weeks back, illustrating the story and how they were piecing together my abuse of him. I kept my head down and got out of there.

Despite the constant uncertainty and fear of my future, I had to return to London and get my life in order. I need to start doing the school run and working out my next moves. While my lawyer was pushing ahead with challenging the caution, my other advisors were asking me to halt it, and I wondered what his thoughts were on the matter. He replied simply, 'It depends how much your reputation means to you.' I didn't need to consider that for long. 'It means the world to me,' I said, and that was that. I was going to forge ahead and proceed regardless of their advice.

I was back, and Jack kept asking if we could meet. I spoke to my mum about wanting to be hardline with him and told her I was being careful in case he sold a story to the papers. However, she reminded me if I did not stand up to him it was like I was still married to him. So I finally told him once and for all that I was going to divorce him, and he must not ring me any more.

He threatened to go to the papers, saying that I had used him as a 'media tool'. It was absurd; I did not need anyone's help in my career, least of all his. And I had never tried to manipulate the papers; rather, I was trying to keep out of them. He was confused and threatening. Daniel rang him to ask him politely to avoid doing that for the sake of our children if nothing else.

The paps were at the bottom of the road every morning, waiting for me to go on the school run. The mornings were dark, so they were using flash photography, and Valentino was getting visibly distressed by it, as was Roman. We all were. It was nothing short of torture. I could do nothing in that moment. Later, I took to Twitter to condemn the press for allowing this, as Valentino was sensitive to flashing lights, and to ask could they please stop. The flash photography did stop overnight, but the cameras were still there.

I called my divorce lawyer, Kay, who got the ball rolling with the legal separation. Jack refused to sign an NDA, citing he would 'never go to the press' and would not agree to any terms of the divorce, no matter how I worded it. There was so much toing and froing, and we were not getting anywhere. In my therapy session I explored letting the argument go and what my options might be. I realised that I could stay separated for the next two years, then the marriage would be dissolved. So I opted for that. Why was I paying to row with this guy? I would never see the money he owed me anyway, and I was desperate to move on.

Despite calling time on the relationship, I also had to go through a mourning process. I had been in love, I thought, but I would never forget anything that had passed, and I was depressed and trying to make sense of what had happened. I read a book on toxic men and what their traits were. I was trying to find the answers through therapy and books, but I was still drinking, and I had nobody around me at the time who was deep enough to be on a level with me.

Then I was suddenly contacted by a blast from the past. Matt's brother Adam messaged me to see how I was. We reconnected, and it was beautiful to talk with someone who had known me as a kid, who knew who I was and did not want anything from me. He came over, and I told him everything.

My professional commitments were still in play, and I had a series of pre-recorded *Let's Do Lunch* Christmas shows airing. Some people on Twitter were incensed that a toxic husband-beater like me was given airtime. My confidence was on the floor. Still, MotoGP was on the cards, and BT still wanted me to sign up. They didn't seem to care about the news reports. I knew it wasn't right but I got talked into it: 'It's a great opportunity,' 'You'll be great, we'll look after you.' All the things I had heard before. And fearing I would never work again, I went against all my instincts and agreed to sign.

I convinced myself that I would learn on the job, and over the winter I educated myself on the riders and the sport's history. But it was hard to remember all of it, putting tons of pressure on myself. The MotoGP fans were hammering me on social media. People were seemingly more angry at me for taking the role than they were about me apparently beating up my husband. In their eyes, this was a bigger crime. It was crazy.

But these people were the least of my worries. It was now evident that the production did not want me either, but because it was the channel's decision they couldn't do much about it except make it clear they would not help me in any way that had been promised.

The first race was in Qatar, and the show was a shambles. We had a technical fault and talkback had gone down – we could not even hear each other speak. It was overwhelming, and I froze. James Toseland was my saviour over this time; he protected and covered me from the barrage of abuse I was getting, when even the subtle disrespect from the guests was evident. I made myself ill with it and wanted out. I had only just been through my own personal suffering, and now I was subjected to it at work. The channel was asking me not to pull out, saying we would do the show from the BT Sports studio and patch through to the races. It was more controlled, so I could cope with what was happening, but yet again the production company were being unhelpful, saying stupid things to me in my ear when we were on air and generally being wankers. I was distraught, and after only four races I broke my contract. Again, BT begged me to not pull out, but it was no good, I had to listen to my gut and get out of there. It was only the second time in my life that I have pulled a contract. My mental health was in tatters, I was living in fear of every race, and my nerves were in shreds. I had to save myself from it all and grin and bear the loss of a decent income and some financial security.

Fortunately, another opportunity came into my life then in the shape of *I'm a Celebrity, Get Me Out of Here*, the show I had turned down a few months ago. Once I had negotiated them up to what I thought it was worth, I agreed and we agreed that I was to enter the jungle the coming winter and must not tell a soul.

Despite this, my reputation was tarnished, and while I was getting some TV work offers on top of *I'm a Celeb*, the better-paid and longer-term endorsement deals were not flowing. So a new friend I had met at the gym suggested I set up a website to promote my thoughts and what I was into and doing. My friend pointed out that my record in the media was so bad it would help that I had a platform to counterbalance it and explain the truth. It was a fantastic idea, but it would cost a chunk of money to set up, and I only had a bit left in the savings account that I was too scared to touch. We were still living in the big flat, and moving felt like an impossible task, as I did not want to disrupt the kids' lives further than I had to. So my friend lent me the money to set up the site and get it going.

They were right, the narrative in the papers needed a reality check, and the website was an exciting way to do that. So I got interviews with some inspirational people I knew and was a fan of and got stuck into writing and coming up with content. I found myself demonstrating a skill set I didn't realise I had, and I was enjoying the positive environment I was creating for myself.

My private life was messy after Jack. I was clawing my way back to some kind of horizon, hiding all my pain and money struggles from the kids – mostly successfully – and I got into silly relationships and mild flirtations here and there. I wasn't respecting myself very well, doing daft things, sleeping with the wrong people and just not respecting myself. I was swerving toxic liars one minute and making a beeline for them the next, just going with desire, not my instincts, or just because I was drunk enough. I decided to never introduce anybody to my children ever again. My relationships would be conducted separately. I was in defence mode and subconsciously seeking unavailable people because I thought if I didn't get close they could not hurt me. That's utter bullshit, of course, but I had to find that out the hard way.

My image was morphing into a more sexy vibe, and Gary suggested I shoot a calendar for the following year. We shot it in Mallorca at my friend Sam's house; it was a fantastic creative process, and I enjoyed being involved. I looked super glam and sexy, but they were just glamorous pics of me; they weren't *me*. In addition, men were starting to be very inappropriate with me because of my strong and sexy image, and I was getting explicit messages from men thinking weird things about me just because they saw some of my flesh. 'I would ruin you' was a common threat. It was an eye-opener and a significant study on a particular strain of straight men, but it also made me uncomfortable and sometimes scared.

Back in the *FHM* days there was no social media, so you would never have to listen or be subjected to what men thought of you or wanted to do to you once your photos were out there. On a very early appearance on *This Morning*, right at the beginning of my TV career, Richard Madeley had asked, after showing a series of sexy images of me in men's mags, if I ever thought about what the readers thought of me and, worse, what they were doing with the pics. I simply replied that they were just glamorous pics of me and that what men chose to do with them was not my business. I was twenty-eight years old at the time, and had been photographed in a million different ways since I was seventeen, but now I was forty-four years old, and the heterosexual male attitudes were more out in the open and dangerously close through social media.

I tried to put it out of my mind; I was off to do the jungle show. Adam came with me as my escort, although I didn't get to hang out with him because I was in the show right until the very end. It was a great experience. It felt like a holiday – no computers, no commitments, no decisions to make. It was bliss. Being told what to do and where to be was way more manageable than my actual life. I loved living small, with few possessions, and logically, despite the risks, I knew nothing would kill me. I really took to sleeping outdoors, too, and I enjoyed some of the other campmates' company even though others drove me quietly mad. I was all out and being myself. However they edited it was up to the production team – I didn't care. I was an excellent mediator when required; I cooked, did my tasks with conviction, and played the game. Hunger was the only real challenge; with my appetite, it was a painful gnawing that I tried to ignore. Not easy. During the show I got very close to Tinchy Stryder. He and I shared a private language, and I washed his clothes when he asked me if it was okay because he did not know how to do it or didn't want to. Either way, I did it in exchange for some spare pairs of socks and bits and pieces he was acquiring from campmates that were leaving. I loved him. Our little deal and secret code were weirdly unnoticed in camp and not used on the show.

I used my logic to not think about the boys, because it wouldn't help. They were in good hands with their father, so I could get on with the job, which required me to be myself and live in the moment. As I crossed the bridge out of the jungle after coming third, I noticed Adam wasn't there to greet me. I knew something was up.

Moments after my chat with Ant and Dec, I was handed a phone. It was my PR agent on the other end. He told me that on the first day of the show, three weeks ago, Jack had sold a huge story about me, even allowing himself to be photographed for it.

The press, I would imagine, would have rung him and said I was going into the jungle and that I would be telling my side of things and it would be best to get his side out first, and I guess he took the bait. But I could be wrong. The fact is, I did not speak about him or say his name once. In fact, I'd stopped using his name entirely in my real life. For me, it was the equivalent of saying Voldemort. I was unnerved and hurt, but underneath it all I felt pity for him. What a desperate thing to do. Deep down, I knew that would always be his weapon against me, the threat from the beginning, and he proved my instinct right. I have never read the piece and never will.

Despite the negativity from Jack and the press, my appearance in the jungle had actually helped some women feel empowered and inspired, and for that I was grateful. Women were celebrating me when I got home. One woman even told me I had given her the fuel she needed to leave her husband after years of an unhappy marriage. I was thrilled. I was getting to help people, and it felt good.

I have always been a woman's woman. I do like some men, but my heart is with my tribe. No one knows what it is like to be a woman but women, and that's a fact. You can be an ally, and thank God for them, but ultimately we must fight our battles and continue trying to be heard. No one will do it for us, nor should we expect them to. We must do it for ourselves.

On the outside, things were fine, work was coming in, and I looked like I was back in control, and I almost convinced myself that I was okay. Then I would get drunk and realise I wasn't. I was about to turn forty-five, and my libido had become a constant torment, but I wasn't up for random encounters. I had done that and I had just felt soiled and worthless every time, they just made me sad, and in the cold sober light of day they were fruitless and were making me ill. I was often introduced to people by friends, so they were not 'strangers', but still it was just not me.

Adam was a constant in my life; I shared everything with him, which was good for me, particularly as he never judged me. I talked to him about exploring giving up drinking, and he agreed it was a good idea and helped me talk to someone he knew who had been sober for years. I went for a walk on the Heath, sat on a bench, spoke about my drinking unguardedly to this man and let it all out. I talked about my behaviour and patterns around booze, and this wonderful guy was supportive and listened without judgement. I felt inspired.

Then my landlord decided he was moving back into my flat, so I finally had to vacate, and in all honesty it was a welcome relief. I needed to move away from Hampstead and needed to be in the catchment area of Tino's next education setting, and Roman was old enough now to get himself to school. It was all change, but it was well needed. So we moved to Golders Green, to live amongst a Hasidic Jewish community. Nobody knew who I was. There were no paps. I loved the place and started to feel 'normal'.

I was still drinking to help me mix with people, but sometimes I would take it too far and make mistakes. I could go months and months at a time and then relapse and get back on it again. I was, however, more off the booze than on it. I was high functioning, keeping the drinking from the kids and physically handling it, but my mental state was suffering.

I was managing to work, though, and was meeting some interesting people – even my childhood idol Boris Becker, who I asked for a photograph. He then invited me to watch some games at Wimbledon in his Centre Court seats. I was pinching myself and tearful. I love Wimbledon and the joy I feel on the Centre Court – the privilege I feel – is intense. As a little girl, it might as well have been Mars, in that there had never seemed the slightest possibility I'd be able to go there, but there I was with my hero.

I was also in love with someone, an 'on-and-off' scenario that had further frayed my heart; I vacillated between being in exqui-site pleasure in his company and being in exquisite pain when we were apart. Our chemistry was off the chart and our connec-tion was deep, but it would never happen. I wasn't in the greatest space anyway, and I thought he could make it all better, save me emotionally, but I eventually realised that job of healing was mine and mine alone.

I was travelling back and forth to Majorca to see my friend Sam, with whom I could share all my troubles and secrets. These trips were my downtime, my breather, my confessional, when I could just let go. Where once Sam had lived in a secluded part of the island, she now had an expansive 180-degree view down into the local town. My thoughts were, if we could see it, it could see us, so I did feel a little vulnerable about relaxing completely when she moved to this house, but I kept pushing my ever-present paranoia to one side. But on one day, the last of my holiday, we sat on the terrace overlooking the view, drinking wine and having the odd puff of weed, and we talked, cried, laughed and chilled. When I woke the next day to fly home I started to feel that I had been careless, and then I experienced that crashing worry that I might have been photographed, which spooked me.

I knew the press would have a field day with an image like that; I could write the piece myself, so well versed was I in their limited vocabulary. But, as ever, the fear that it would impact work was real. I had to fly home, and I admonished myself all the way back, praying that I wasn't coming home to a shit storm about drugs, and I beat myself up for days for letting my guard down. Finally, when the photos did not emerge, I realised it had all been in my head, which shook me. I could not live like this any more. I had the foresight to see where things could and would happen, and now the PTSD had finally caught up with me, and so this time, without hitting an actual rock bottom, I could fight my way back in private. I vowed to not live like this any more.

Yet again, I returned to the same psychiatrist, who finally sent me to an addiction specialist. She was great and started to put some good reading material in front of me, Maya Angelou and Brené Brown – brilliant, strong and articulate messaging that spoke to me and gave me some fight. Finally, I saw another way of being. I was very focused, and for the first time the action of abstaining was becoming easy

I also went back and forth to LA, visiting a friend who took me to AA meetings. I found these very interesting, I sympathised and empathised with people's stories but didn't speak; I just listened. I was interested in the steps and realised I had done many of them already. I had been cleaning up, apologising and making amends with people along the way, too. I felt addicted to my sobriety. And I found it interesting that everybody would ask me how I was doing it, then tell me they wouldn't be able to. Everyone said that to me. So I realised that most people I was meeting actually had a serious drinking problem.

I was feeling blessed, and opportunities were coming in. I became the new 'voice of Graham' for the *Blind Date* rebooted TV show with Paul O'Grady at the helm, and I shot a third Boddingtons advert. Sadly, I wasn't impressed with the finished cut. I was told I would have a say in the edit, but that was not honoured and, as always, my suggestions were ignored. The result was a massive disappointment to me; it was not funny.

Blind Date became complicated too. I was asked if I would make a visible appearance on the show for the Christmas Special. The 'ask' was that I be wheeled onto the set and jump out of a cake as a surprise to the audience. I was dumbfounded. I could not believe they thought I would be up for such shite. Treating me like some kind of 'showgirl' at my age. They told me that Paul had agreed it would be a brilliant idea and that everyone would be in fancy dress. I declined. Later, at the studio, I went to see Paul in his dressing room. He was outraged as he hadn't even agreed to the fancy dress, let alone backed the idea of me jumping out of a cake. I was equally outraged, and we bitched, moaned and had to laugh at the absurdity of this ridiculous industry.

The press was still writing total shit about me – getting a grain of something and turning it into something much bigger. Around this time, private photos were hacked from my phone, which I had taken and were meant for my lover's eyes only. I was devastated. It's true that my shoots for *FHM* and my calendar weren't that far away from them, but they were still private photographs. I was humiliated and angry. The press announced it, and although they weren't allowed to print the pics themselves, the article drove many more people to search them out and take a look.

My first year of sobriety was empowering, but I was still vulnerable in the industry. My agent was encouraging me to appear on game shows to remind people I was still on the scene. He believed they would be harmless, good payers and decent exposure, so I agreed to appear on *The Chase* with Bradley Walsh, who I knew and trusted. The quick-fire element to the questioning was problematic for me; I was never comfortable being put on the spot with general knowledge, even though I had form at pub quizzes. The last thing I heard Bradley advise was that if we didn't know the answer we should say 'pass' and move on to save time. I logged this information and then did precisely that; panicked and passed on everything, even the things I knew. I did not trust myself and was too stressed to find the information in my brain. The press wrote some shit about me upsetting Bradley, which was not true. I have always been a fan of that man and his magic, and from what he tells me he likes me too, but the whole thing was stressful.

I was also asked to be on the guessing panel of *Through the Keyhole* with the character Keith Lemon at the helm. I had just returned from a five-day break to Mallorca with my mate and I was feeling relaxed and happy and thought it might be an okay gig. I had been on *Celebrity Juice* some years before, as Gino had asked me to appear on it. I had never watched it, but I knew it was risqué, and the experience had been challenging – I'd felt at that time that I had to be mildly inebriated during that experience to get through it. However, I thought the sexual content would be absent from the 'keyhole' show as this was for families on a Saturday night, so I assumed I would be safe from Keith's innuendoes. I was wrong.

His opening line in introducing me was to ask if 'my arsehole smelled of flowers?' He commented that he imagined me as Pocahontas and that all my clothes came off. He used me to entertain the big crowd, and I was trapped. If I left, it would make the papers that I had walked, so I was frozen to my seat and panicking because of my feelings of claustrophobia, unable to get out of a situation, and I wanted to cry. I chose to minimise the impact by enduring it all, which of course did not minimise the effect on me.

By the time I got home I was in pieces. I could not sleep and I cried all night. I had been used for entertainment value and I had had enough. No respect had been shown towards me, and nobody had stopped the behaviour either. I had one camera locked on me the whole night that captured everything. I would be devastated to see any footage of me that night broadcast. The next day I rang my agents and told them what had happened. They told me they would ring production, but I decided to deal with it myself.

I asked for the final cut on all my shots so that I did not look upset, angry or out of my depth at any time during the show. Any expression out of context would show my displeasure, which would have defeated the object of my 'appearance' in the first place. The production team agreed to my terms. They told me that I was the only person to ever complain, as if somehow that would make a difference to me.

No one would have known when it was aired, and no one would have an inkling of my opinion that night, but the experience is forever etched in my memory. In what world is that considered entertainment? The industry was the pits, and I wanted out. I vowed then and there that I would never appear on television again unless I was actually 'presenting' a show, and I made this very clear to my agent.

I was also noticing problematic relationships I was having with women. I could only see the good in these women and wanted to help them with their problems, and there were people who also tried to help me, but they used me to elevate themselves, and when I took their good advice, ran with their ideas and started to thrive, their jealousy kicked in and the friendships would implode. Their jealousy would be exposed, and I would have to call time on these relationships. It seemed like I was in a pattern of meeting people who deep down did not want the best for me.

I started to like my own company, fully pursue my interests and enjoy myself. I found solace in the movies, the theatre, and going to art galleries, and I read voraciously. I was getting well. My sobriety was peeling away layers, my inner voice was becoming stronger, and more importantly I was starting to listen to it. I felt it was a calling to go to the motherland, to travel to Rajasthan and stand on the soil of my ancestors. I knew this would be very healing for me, so I began to look at travel packages. I asked Adam if he was interested in coming with me. When he said yes, I was delighted. I needed to get away, regroup, catch my breath and reconnect with myself, and he was the perfect companion. So we booked the holiday and flights. The date we were leaving was 1 May, which marked a year to the day of my sobriety.

Chapter 15

India was all I expected and more. I'd been told to brace myself for the heat, the smell, the poverty, the noise and the traffic by numerous people; it seemed to be the stock line that people spouted, but when I landed at Delhi airport and took one look around me, I loved it.

We headed straight into traffic in a cab. Horns blared relentlessly, and the hustle and bustle of the hot evening hummed. I wound down the window and took it all in. It was thrilling to be there. As we journeyed to our hotel and saw more of Indian life, instead of feeling like I had to brace myself for anything I instantly succumbed to it. I was in sensory heaven and emotional harmony. This was India, and it felt like home.

We didn't indulge in five-star travel, nor were we backpacking. Instead, we stayed in some quirky independent hotels with their different charms and challenges, and each stop was an adventure. Adam reminded me we should use the trip to acknowledge my year of sobriety, which I agreed to do. I was not in the habit of patting myself on the back for anything, and I knew it was an unhealthy stance that I needed to shake.

We got up early for a train to Agra on our first day to see the Taj Mahal. I had a lifelong ambition to see it in the flesh since staring at the beautiful miniature model in Nanna's showcase, and I felt this trip was for all of my family that never returned.

Adam and I talked to a guy on the train, and he asked us where we were heading. I told him that my mum was from Gangapur, and we weren't sure if it was possible to fit it into our itinerary. So we all looked on the map, and he showed us which stage of the journey would have a reasonable detour that wouldn't put us too far off schedule. It was set, and it felt heartening to contemplate.

There is so much politics around the Anglo-Indians; some see themselves as English, and some are understandably confused by this dual identity. The fact is that Anglo-Indians are both English and Indian, no matter how it is interpreted by anybody or what alliances they chose to make with either country. Roots are roots, and they/we are both. I found the people in India to be just wonderful – there wasn't a bad attitude in sight no matter where we went, no matter what the situation. There were high vibrations everywhere, and I love it and them.

Travelling with Adam was a joy, too. Everything was easy, with no pressure. We went with the flow. I didn't have to try with him. We talked and talked, and I cried and cried. One minute I was talking through trauma and in floods of tears, the next minute I had tears of laughter pouring down my face. Adam is the only person I laugh with like that, and I revel in it. It happens nearly every time I see him, and it's always something so silly, with impeccable timing.

I was also starting to feel more grounded there than I ever had before. My routine was to wake up and feel grateful to be there. I knew we were having an adventure – and an adventure of a lifetime. We experienced such beauty, marvelled at the incredible architecture, learned about history and crossed the country on long journeys to see India in its humble and majestic glory. The whole experience was a feast for the heart and soul, and I was experiencing a new kind of presence. I began to see things in detail, from a flash of bird flight streaking across the car window to the echoing sanguine worship of morning prayer. I was tuning in and waking up.

I shared some of my journey on Instagram, and it was lovely to see people responding well with the possibility of them also visiting India. I was opening up this beautiful country to people who may never have thought of going there as a holiday destination, and it made me really happy. I loved the food; eating spicy and delicious curries every day was bliss, and I am never not in the mood for a curry. The sunsets and sunrises nourished me and brought me a sense of inner peace and calm. This mood was taking over and taking root. My soul searching revealed all the blessings I had and the guardian angels who'd always been there for me. I realised that even in my darkest days I could find the light, or it had found its way to me. I became grounded and moved by the country's spiritual pull.

The day arrived to travel to Gangapur. It was an India we hadn't seen before; the heat was intense, and we weren't sure we were in the right place. We pulled over to get a Coke from a roadside vendor and asked for directions. There was rubbish all over the roads, street bonfires and pigs foraging through the burning debris. It looked like a post-apocalyptic scene in a movie; it was unreal yet at the same time very centring.

We were not far from our destination and we soon found Gangapur railway station. I jumped out to get a picture, then we followed a quieter road up to an opening that flattened out to a gated community. It was an estate surrounded by a picket fence and looked almost deserted. It was the colony of my family. I was finally here.

It was a peaceful spot, only a stone's throw from the city centre that we had just passed through, but we could hear nothing of it on the wind. A small Catholic church welcomed our arrival, and we got out to take a closer look. The churchwarden told us it was closed, but I told her my mum had lived here when she was a child, and where I came from, and what a shame it was not to be able to go inside. She told me to wait, then went off to get the priest. He came out and I explained again why I was there. He was very accommodating and kindly opened up the church for us to go and have a look.

It was simple and beautiful, designed for a small congregation. I asked if it might be possible if he could see if there were any records of marriages, deaths or baptisms connected to my family. So he took us into a side room, and I had to do a bit of maths on dates and was messaging Mum for info back in England. They handed me a book and I started to scroll through the pages, and there they were, my Nana and Grandad's names with the baptism details of my mum. Seeing them registered all those years ago in their hand was incredible. I could imagine my beautiful Nan and Grandad proudly signing the book to celebrate their firstborn. It was so incredibly powerful and, of course, I cried. Adam took pictures to mark the moment.

We walked around the grounds, and Adam hung back to give me some space, always thoughtful and kind. I found the 'institute' – the location of so many family stories. I didn't know the exact position of the family home, and quite a few houses were derelict, while other were still lived in. It must have been wonderful at its peak, with all the families and friends having fun in this little community, and I could start to quantify the loss that my family may have felt when they came to England.

I felt a deep love for my mum and all the family, and I was in floods of tears. Before I left, I stood there and took in the heat and the sounds, wanting to take in what they felt, smelled and experienced all those years ago. I know it looked different, but the elements surrounding the place were the same, and I wanted my body to log it all and connect with their experience. As I stared out of the back of the car, it felt like a missing piece in my heart had been filled, and I realised what a healing experience it had been.

I was connected, and it felt incredible. It was like I was putting pieces of myself together, giving me a kind of wisdom. India opened my portal for more self-discovery, and I will forever be grateful for that.

The energy of India reflected my heart and soul, and I felt set free.

I was a million miles from being watched, photographed and stalked. I was under the radar and enjoying my life. We travelled by train and car and visited many extraordinary places with incredible views. We went on safari in Ranthambore, hung out in Jaipur, travelled to Pushkar and marvelled at the bathing ghats at the lake. We took a steam train journey in Deogarh and finally to Udaipur, taking a boat trip on the lake. We feasted on curries while overlooking the fruit bats swooping and diving over Lake Pichola, which was our evening entertainment.

Towards the end of the trip, after soul-searching about love and relationships and the weight of unrequited love, I had an epiphany during one of our very last breakfasts in India. I suddenly realised what I've been doing with my personal relationships all these years. I had ignored all the red flags whenever I was having sex with someone I liked, and if the sex was good I would not engage with the warnings, not acknowledge them because I enjoyed the sex more. I realised all this behaviour was toxic for me, and I decided that I needed to be celibate. I decided I would date with caution in future, get to know people first, and see how it went. That way I could get a measure of someone from the get-go and work out what they wanted. When Adam came to join me at the table, I told him of my revelation. He was supportive and agreed it was a good idea and it was definitely worth a go.

Saying goodbye to India was tough, but the growth I had experienced both spiritually and mentally on my trip was the greatest gift it had given me and I could take everywhere. I just had to work out how I could take these lessons home and make sense of my silly, senseless job. I had to find some deep meaning in my life and make some changes.

Chapter 16

I still had some vocal audio pick-ups to do for *Blind Date,* but it all felt embarrassing. What was I doing? It was just for money, which was fine, but it was unfulfilling in the extreme.

I was recording with my exec producer Michelle, and we chatted about what happened to me in India. I told her I had started to find myself and was struggling to work out how to assimilate my spiritual awakening into my ridiculous career. It felt brave and necessary to tell my boss that I thought my work was trivial, but she was brilliant and totally understood. She told me she was a meditation teacher and had studied with Deepak Chopra. She had had a similar realisation years ago. She had had a high-flying TV job and had suffered burnout. She suggested I enrol in her course, so I rang Adam and asked him if he was interested in coming.

It was only a few evenings, but it was the start of my journey to understanding myself in spirit and not attaching myself to every thought I had, and that I was not my body or my mind, I was pure energy. I took to it straight away. In fact, the first time

I meditated alone, I suddenly felt all my energy in my root chakra and nearly had an orgasm. It was powerful, and I suddenly understood what tantric sex might be about. So the next day I rang Michelle to ask her if that was common, and she laughed 'No, it's not!'

My friend Caroline also got me into hot yoga. My first class was hilarious and ridiculous, I was so uncoordinated and unable to make all the moves. I loved how strong you had to be, though, and it was next level, with 90-minute lessons of intense, crazy poses, but I just loved it.

The yoga, combined with my meditation, was getting me into a better space. I was calmer and slowly found some peace in my life. I was looking for a route out of my work situation. At the time, I was voicing a reality TV show that was easy work – harmless but mindless. I was working with a fun producer and doing the recording with her, which made it bearable. I stopped playing the game and instead shared with people who I was. As a result, I was living more authentically for the first time.

I was still open to dating, despite my vow of celibacy, and I met a guy locally. He seemed nice, and I agreed to go for dinner with him. I told him where I was at, and that I was looking for friendships first, getting to know people properly before developing physical relationships with them. He seemed to get it and displayed an understanding. After dinner, he offered to give me a lift home, so I said yes. Then when we pulled up outside my house, he tried to kiss me. I was horrified. I pushed him away and asked, 'Did you not hear anything I was just telling you?' His reply was: 'You can't look like that and expect me not to try.' 'Yeah, I actually can, dickhead,' I thought. I could not get out of his car fast enough. It was another brilliant lesson about what it was that I wanted: a man to at least hear me. Was that too much to ask?

The celibacy thing was brilliant, an experiment that was good for me. I could observe male behaviour, which gave me a brilliant insight into men and who they fundamentally were, and I had control for the first time over my libido. It was a win-win. The year was perfect for me; no longer would I be used by anybody; my respect for myself shot up as my respect for men diminished.

Alan and I were now doing the Saturday morning slot on Radio 2 for the summer seasons while Graham Norton took his break from the show. Alan was a friend, I could connect with him away from the business and talk about art, books, travel and deeply silly things, and I told him *everything*.

Our producer Malcolm Prince was an absolute joy, too. He understood what I could bring to the show and could see my value. However, I struggled with the show's mechanics. Getting in and out of records was tough, with hard counts and all the technical stuff I didn't want to do. I was just awful at it, so Alan had that covered, but sometimes Malcolm gave me a stab at it even though I would complain. My nerves would grip me, and I always fucked it, much to the amusement of us all.

I did, however, love the interviews. I loved researching the guests and coming up with questions. It felt great to be part of an uplifting, giggle-inducing show, and it was as much of a tonic for me as it was for our listeners. Of course, we had our critics, which is standard, but we were fun and lighthearted, and the fans were terrific. Our audience shared their special moments and the daft stories of their lives, which ultimately added to the fun. They were an absolute hoot.

I was now practising yoga intermittently with the gym. As I was getting older, I wanted a combination of flexibility, balance and strength, and it worked. I was forty-eight, in tip-top shape, feeling good, grounded, focused and desperate to change my professional life. My friend Caroline and I talked about it at length, and she suggested we start an online magazine together for women over forty. It instantly appealed to me. My first thought was that we should use models over forty, too, as we were so underrepresented in the mainstream mags, and I wanted to make a change. I knew someone who could do the tech side and build it for us while we got the content together.

We all decided to create a bi-monthly, online, flickable magazine, but first we needed a name. I wanted it to be something that represented me; I was speaking my truth and had always been forthright with my opinion. I like to tell it like it is and call things out if they're bullshit, and I wanted the magazine to reflect that. So, over a brainstorm one day, a colleague said, 'What about "Frank"?' 'Oh my God, it's perfect,' I said. Caroline wasn't sure of the name at first and needed time to think about it, but I was itching to get going. Luckily she agreed to the name, and *The Frank Magazine* was born.

I realised a strong creative vision and instinctively knew how to bring it together. So I threw myself into it with every fibre of my being.

My sister came down to see me and opened me up to some good things to watch on telly, as she always does. *The Trip* was one of them, and I thought it was bloody fantastic. Steve Coogan was exquisitely funny, and he piqued my interest. He was my age, intelligent, Northern and funny and I liked him a lot. I talked to a few close friends about him, including Alan. So when

Steve invited Alan to the press screening of *Stan and Ollie*, Alan asked me if I wanted to be his plus one. I was so chuffed I might get to meet him, and despite the fact I'd already seen the film I was more than happy to see it again.

After the event, I rang our mutual friend, John Thompson, to get him to ask Steve if I could have his number with a view to going for dinner. John said yes, and so did Steve. So I messaged him and asked him out.

He was charming, a total gentleman, silly, fun and super smart. Steve knew his worth, had no qualms about flexing his vast intellect and felt no need to play down his creative talents, considerable as they were, and I admired him. He possessed a truth I hadn't ever seen before, making me a little nervous, and I liked it and really liked him.

It was in the paper before we really knew each other, and I had barely told anyone about it. Even my mum messaged me to ask if it was true. The narrative about me romantically focused on meeting the 'one'. I have never thought of people like that. I don't believe in the 'one'. I believe in experiences and connecting with people's souls without expectation. I believe in being with a person until it stops working for either of you for whatever reasons and you part ways amicably. If people want to compromise, that's cool too, but speaking personally, I do not consider romantic relationships the be-all and end-all of my life.

My time with Steve taught me I wanted to be around creatives; I needed that stimulation. I'd often had dinner with men over the years, professionally and romantically, and I internally would be begging them to please tell me something I didn't already know. But my intuition guided me to a different kind of person; unbeknownst to Steve, he helped me locate my sapiosexual inclination and to know what I deserve. He's a genius. He deserves even more recognition than he gets, and I bloody love him.

But I was so fed up with having my private life plastered all over the papers; I was just so tired of it. I had no privacy. The magazine, however, was a brilliant addition to my life. I was pulling together all my skills. Skills I didn't even know I possessed; they were just pouring out of me. I was getting interviews, arranging shoots, booking models, talking to stylists and sourcing writers, all with a budget of a big fat zero, and I was getting shit done. We were all about female empowerment and wanted to promote women achieving great things in their forties and celebrating their achievements.

Regarding the 'look' of the magazine, I had definite ideas within our budget of nothing. I looked at spreads and knew what to do with them. I had a good eye for looking at a page and knowing precisely what it needed. I could see the inaccuracies of things and could use my innate knowledge of how to make things look good. I started to get excited about font sizes and spacing. The perfecting of the pages really got me going.

It was great but it was exhausting. The colleague most closely involved patiently listened to all my notes and directions. It was hours and hours of intense work. I was delighted at the skill set that had just been unearthed. I was ensconced in my new role and loved it.

We ended up with a two-hundred-page magazine because the content was always coming in, and I never wanted to sit on anything. If I had it, it was getting published. I was having meetings and reaching out to brands for advertising space. Nobody was being paid, but we were building our business; it was hard graft but, most importantly, great fun. I felt like I'd found my calling, and to discover another layer of myself and something that I was good at gave me confidence, not knocked it out of me. The magazine was launched, and the hard work continued, but I was definitely on the right path.

Chapter 17

Having a new role in my work life was meaningful and felt nourishing. I felt less attached to show business now, and my extraction from its financial dependence was in motion.

I was still enjoying my radio show when Malcolm announced that he had managed to organise a trip to Universal Studios in Florida to broadcast some shows. I was excited to travel, never one to miss an opportunity to get on a flight, but I was not a big lover of theme parks. In fact, I hated rollercoaster rides. I had only ever been on the Big Dipper at Blackpool pleasure beach and kept my head down, eyes closed and prayed for my life through every rickety twist, turn and dip. There was no question that I would be doing any of the rides, and I made it crystal clear that that was not on the cards.

We had to apply for work visas, which was a bit of a faff. Alan and I went to the American visa office and sat it out. When it came to answering the forms it said, 'Have you ever been arrested or convicted for any offence or crime, even though subject of a pardon, amnesty or other similar action?' So, of course, I put yes. When I got to the counter, I told the clerk the caution had been revoked, and it was established that I had to obtain proof of that before the visa would be granted. The clock was ticking on our departure date, so this was another added stress for production. We got the paperwork in on time, but what a palaver.

The first day in Florida consisted of going to the park and recording audio for our first show. Malcolm asked me if I was up for going on 'The Revenge of the Mummy', a mild ride, not a big-time rollercoaster, reassuring me that I would be fine. So I agreed. It was indoors and high-paced; all I could do was scream like a banshee, throwing me into wild laughter and back again. I was going in any direction and at many speeds in complete darkness; it was bloody scary and exhilarating. Malcolm told me I had nearly deafened him in his headphones; my vocal had gone off the scale. It was a brilliant loss of control and a release that was utterly liberating.

All that said, Alan was up next, and I was not joining him on his ride. This was a serious rollercoaster with an almost vertical drop called 'The Hollywood Rip Ride' – I felt sick just looking at it. Alan and Malcolm were on camera at the front of the carriage, the worst spot or best spot, depending on how you perceive it. Alan's reactions were hilarious and got a shit tonne of views online – over ten million to date.

The show went okay. We managed to get into our groove even though the dynamic and studio setting were very different to home, and that, coupled with the time difference, was interesting. We had some fun audio packages from interviewing Olive Oyl and Sinbad – a career high if you ask me – and some guests in the studio; we talked to astronaut Jon McBride about his adventures in space, which was pretty cool. So it was a mixed bag, but it seemed to work, and I think we got away with it.

I was having breakfast with Alan on our last day and I asked him if he fancied going on the 'Incredible Hulk' ride. He laughed, 'What have you done with Melanie Sykes?' After all the laughs and screams, I was open to tackling the big one. The build-up had been through the water park rides, and I was going on everything. I had never been on a ride where your legs dangled down, previously appalled by the idea of it, so the fact that I was contemplating it was crazy. We got all the team together and off we went. I have just googled the ride, and its opening line is 'Unleash You Inner Hulk', which I'm pretty sure happened to me, and it was liberating. What a total blast.

The things I learned on this trip? That Astronauts, no matter their age, are flirts; I was an undiscovered adrenalin junkie; and that I have a thing for Spiderman. All in all, it was a brilliant, informative and hilarious trip.

Hanging out with Alan was really compelling, too. We were permanently interrupted; people flocked to him, wanted pictures, and praised him. I stood back and watched and sometimes offered to take the photos. I was invisible, and it was fantastic. Alan was very good with people and accommodating, something I've always found hard to do. Most of the time I was approached or called out to when I was alone. I'd stopped agreeing to selfies because I hated the embrace of strangers and the intrusion, the energetic crash into my boundaries and the further scrutiny from casual onlookers.

Once, travelling alone, I woke up on a train with somebody taking my picture, woken by the click of the phone they had forgotten to put on silent. People video me on the underground, and I often try to mentally curl up into balls and hide myself away, so nobody would notice me. It would make long journeys problematic, and being trapped with lots of questions and people staring was a constant threat. I've had to hide on beaches or airports and position myself so I am not seen by British people on holiday. I found normalcy with the locals and people from other countries who had never heard of me. Everyone else behaved like they knew me already; their curiosity and gawping turned me inside out. It was rare that people wanted to speak to me about anything important or on a level. Often people just say 'Boddingtons' and move on. It was baffling; I don't know what I am supposed to do with it. Men come over with children holding pieces of paper for me to sign, and I know the child has no idea who I am. I call this out repeatedly and say, 'How do you know me?' Finally, the kid exposes their parent's intention by saying, 'I don't know, my dad asked me to do it.' It is an absurdity that would be funny if I didn't loathe it so much, and I always feel sorry for the kids.

One summer, I was on an aeroplane off to have a weekend break when the stewardess started handing out the *Sun* newspaper. The man sitting next to me began to flick through the pages, then glanced over his shoulder; I saw, to my horror, that there in the paper was a shot of me on my previous holiday. I had just dived into Lake Como to dunk myself in, and there was a photo of me pulling myself back onboard a boat. I wanted to vaporise. Everybody on the plane had a copy of it except me. With searing discomfort, I stared out the window the entire flight, not daring to go to the loo, not wanting to be recognised, and my mind raced about how the press knew where I had been.

But travel was part of my life. It punctuated my work, sometimes it *was* my work, which meant I had to balance my other work and my parenting with it. But I had other creative outlets in my work. The magazine work was a constant joy, even through the long hours of graft, and the team and I were bonding and having fun.

I was feeling pretty together, had got a handle on my libido, and learned to control and calm my fire. I also processed how much I had been disrespected by men throughout my life. It had occurred at work, at home, on the street and on my phone. The threat was real and everywhere, and my dislike of toxic men was ballooning, but now I was in a better position to protect myself and learning every day, and I felt healthy and happy.

Being there for the children was the constant that kept me going. As always, my boys were terrific and needed my help. The older they got, the more interesting my parenting became. I was there to protect and encourage them but not be pushy. I held strict boundaries and rules that they respected, and I relished my role.

My work was also always interesting; random offers and asks came in regularly. However, I always turned down more than I said yes to. Most things were not suitable, or I had no desire to be involved in low-quality productions or things I deemed dull and could not fake enjoyment of.

During one of my voiceover records for the reality show, my producer told me she was leaving and going to work on a show called *The Great Pottery Throw Down*. I'd seen it advertised but hadn't watched it. Sara Cox wasn't doing the next season, and they were looking for a new presenter. I really didn't want to entertain the idea. She knew I was out of the game, but she still encouraged me to at least think about it.

She said she'd mentioned my name anyway, and the Exec Producer, Sarah, had been interested in meeting me. She thought it might be good to just go and chat with her. I wasn't sure and was almost scared to go into the fray again, but I kept thinking, how toxic could a show centred around potters be? So after I was sent links to watch the last season, I thought maybe it was a lovely show and harmless, and perhaps I might be able to manage what would be required of me. So a meeting was arranged.

Sarah Thomson-Woolley was wonderful, and I warmed to her immediately. I told her about all my problems and how I didn't want to do TV any more. I was terrified of the big pieces to camera and some of the mechanics of making programmes, but on the other hand I always enjoyed appearing on other people's shows where the pressure was off me. I was totally out of practice; I hadn't presented anything for nearly two years, which had brought happiness and I didn't want to jeopardise that.

It was for the same production company that made *The Great British Bake Off* and was respected because of its success. I had appeared on the *Stand Up To Cancer* version of the show for charity, the production was good and the filming had run well. So I allowed myself to explore the idea. A few weeks later, an agreement was set, and I was back in the mix.

We filmed in Stoke-on-Trent for months, and it was all-consuming. I was juggling a lot, the work at the shoot was relentless and intense, and I was nervous much of the time. I had asked if I could go on a potter's wheel before we started filming just so I knew what it felt like, and I was getting used to the layout of the building and the rooms we were filming in to get acclimatised. And because it was working pottery and there was limited space, the judges and I had to share one dressing room, so we had no privacy. Luckily I was sharing with the charming Keith Brymer Jones, who was a massive part of the show's conception, and the wonderful Sue Pryke, who was new to the show like me.

It was an enormous production, everyone was lovely, and I was particularly happy to be working again with a great make-up artist called Sally who I'd been impressed by before, and now could work with properly and have fun with. Still I felt overwhelmed. I was nervous about venturing out, because if I stepped out to get any space somewhere, someone would come up and talk to me and make sure I was okay, when all I wanted was five minutes to breathe and be left alone. So I rarely went to dinner with anyone and did not go to the wrap party either. I couldn't mingle like everyone else seemed to be able to. I just didn't want or need it.

I was on call to go into the studio in case something happened, and I was on pins, worried I would freeze out there and not find the words to articulate what was happening. I felt so watched. And, of course, I was watched; there were cameras everywhere, and I found it challenging. I absolutely loved all the elements of the show and the show itself, but I wasn't sure about myself within it. I was trying to relax as if the cameras weren't there, knowing it would be so much better if I did, but I was still coming across well, luckily. I was interested in the process and mindsets of potters, how creativity flows, and what forms it takes. We had experts who were fascinating characters and who demonstrated detailed and impressive skills. All the potters had a story to tell, wisdom to impart and humour, and I supported them in different ways. They just needed to feel at ease enough to create something good; hopefully, I helped them achieve that.

Again, the pieces to the camera were a massive problem for me. The director helped by breaking them down with me into shots; sometimes they needed it in one go, which I struggled to do. I would have sleepless nights over them before filming, and even though the crew were terrific, kind and patient, I tied myself in knots over remembering words.

I was going to be back on the television in January. I was nervous until I saw the footage when I went in to record the voiceover to pictures, and I could see it looked fantastic. It was well received, and people thoroughly enjoyed it. I was also told that there probably would be another season.

It was Des's birthday, and his wife Jodie had invited me to the house to go and see him. We talked over a bit of cake and a coffee about the past, our Des and Mel days and what was happening in our worlds. Then he and Jodie started talking about maybe getting a show underway to celebrate his life and career. They wondered if I thought it was a good idea.

It sounded like an excellent idea to me. Jodie said they had been thinking about ringing Bradley Walsh, a dear friend of Des's, to see if he could help make this happen. 'I'll do it. I'll get a meeting with Kevin Lygo and chat with him about it,' I said. 'I'm sure he'll be up for it.'

I was about to attend the National Television Awards, and I thought I'd ask the head of ITV about setting up a meeting while I was there. In the run-up to the event I also rang Alan and asked him if he'd walk the red carpet with me, because of how much I loathe going on them – the lights, the flashing cameras, the levels of sound and all manner of sensory overload, all while trying to hold myself together. I needed support, and he agreed that we'd walk together comfortably inside; I said a few hellos to a few people and went to see Kevin in the ITV suite and talked to him briefly about Des and asked if I could get a meeting about a possible documentary. He agreed, and I left.

A few days later, I got my meeting and went down to ITV to have a chat with him further. I told him that Des was frail and how incredible it would be to make a lovely fitting tribute to him and his career before he died instead of cobbling something together last minute. He deserved some recognition now, and it would be fantastic for Des to have a hand in that.

He agreed on the spot, and the programme was commissioned. He asked me to see the head of factuals who, in turn, asked me to speak to ITN Productions. I met with ITN and got the documentary rolling for Des. I was given Executive Producer credit, but for whatever reason I was elbowed out once they'd hooked up with Des, in true TV style, but this wasn't about me, so I let it go.

However, I still had to do a master interview for my talking head bits. They wanted to have some soundbites about how I felt about Des, and this was to be filmed quite late on.

Around the same time I was asked to screen test for a BBC consumer show. I had worked with the producer before, and off the back of my performance on *The Great Pottery Throw Down*, she had asked me to come to do a chemistry test/audition. I didn't want to get into all this TV lark again, but as my agent said, it was money and a harmless show.

So I got the job working with Joanna Page on *Shop Well for Less*. Joanna is absolutely brilliant, and we could let off steam laughing and sharing our crazy work stories; we were on a level and we laughed a lot, and I loved her the more I worked with her. It was a friendly enough format with good intentions, but I'd forgotten how much nonsense went around filming. Essentially, all the setups were fake and staged, and I was required to make it look natural. Joanna and Sally were the only things making it bearable; I wasn't into it.

We did my first day of filming up in Leicester, and then a week later there were rumblings about a virus in China that had been killing people, and it was reported in the news that it had made its way to Britain. We were told that if we came into contact with anybody with symptoms or with the virus itself we had to isolate for fourteen days. I had the magazine cover shoot set up, wondering whether I should pull it, and I also had filming to do up in Leicester. I rang my agent. Was it wise to be filming in people's houses? The news was getting more and more concerning, and he said, 'Oh, it's allright, it's something and nothing, it will blow over.'

So I cracked on and had a wonderful time shooting with the *Frank* team; we talked about the virus but also enjoyed the day's work. Our cover model and I were having a fun chat about men; she told me she was on a dating website for many creatives and beautiful, interesting people, and it was deemed a private members' club for dating. She gave me the lowdown on the site and the background, and I thought it might be worth exploring. So she nominated me, and I was accepted.

That afternoon, on the way up to filming, I got a call from production to say that Joanna's agent had been on and she had pulled out because of the news of the virus. I was relieved and could not wait to go home, but unfortunately the next day I found out I had been in contact with someone with the symptoms, and so I had to isolate. My children had to stay put with Daniel. For now, I was on my own.

It was an interesting fourteen days; I realised more things were slowing down as the news feed was ramping up, and my incarceration started to feel like a blessing. Of course I was concerned by the death toll and the stories of suffering, but I was happy in my little flat and world. I didn't have to go anywhere, I didn't have to be anyone, I didn't have to talk to anyone, and I was in my element.

I was exercising and doing yoga. I was cooking, working on the magazine, reading tons, and even started an online book club with Simon Savidge, who my agent had put me in touch with as he knew what an avid reader I was and thought we would get on very well. He thought we would be a good match. Books are Simon's business, so he was a great guide and a blast to work with. I found it joyful to be discussing books in public. Initially nervous, I started to relax and have fun with Simon, and people were enjoying our conversations. We did quite a few video recordings online months before actually meeting in the flesh, but by then I felt like I already knew him, and it was brilliant.

I was also dabbling on my new dating app. I wasn't able to actually meet anybody in the flesh, so it felt safe and just a bit of fun. It asked to choose an age range and type, so I put creative, and the age question was interesting. I like to know the age of people because it helps me understand their cultural touchstones. Regarding the question of age preference, I gauged opinions from my younger friends, who were in their twenties and thirties, and my much older friends – people in their eighties and nineties. So I set the age range at twenty-five to fifty-plus.

I spoke more to people from other countries who did not know who I was already. I was talking to a guy in the States, and then this dude popped up in my DMs who I had liked. His introduction was hilarious, and I proceeded to indulge him. He was fantastic, funny and totally a pain in the arse. He amused me, and I liked him. His name was Mathieu Kassovitz; he is an actor, a director, a writer, an activist, a full-on French rebel and a total hoot. We had the most hilarious conversations, and he challenged me about my ideas about everything and loosened me up. The sexual chemistry lit me up, too. I had become relatively rigid in my thinking without realising it, browbeaten by the so-called rules of my industry about what women were allowed and not allowed to do. I explained my suffering and lack of private life, and he gave me advice. He was so experienced, and slightly older than me; what he said was all gold dust. We FaceTimed and chatted. It helped to pass the lockdown time, and we had fun planning when we might be able to meet.

I was watching the news religiously, keeping up to speed with what was going on, and sticking to the rules rigidly. I was studying politicians and became interested in world politics and different thinkers. The narrative was mixed and confusing as time passed, and then Dominic Cummings went on a drive that changed everything. I was angry and cried for days. I was incensed that these jokers were dictating terms and thinking they were excluded from them. I was devastated, and that's when I started to really wake up.

Once the kids were back with me, the time in the flat during lockdown was good on the whole; I was cooking, baking, running my magazine, and ensuring Valentino was doing online classes with his school. Roman was waiting for his A-level results and hoping to actually be able to attend university. Of course, we were all a bit stir-crazy at times, but, thankfully, never all at once. The kids were now young adults and the flat had become small. Once I had to get out and go for a short drive just to scream in the car. All my frustration came out. Afterwards I rang a friend and cried for a bit, pulled myself together, felt a million times better, and then returned home. I have since heard of scream therapy, and I totally get it. I, at that time, found it through my instincts, which, when listened to, have usually served me well.

As restrictions eased, more opportunities arose. When travel opened up, I got a train to finally meet Matthieu and hang out for a while. Work was starting up again, too. I was approached by a publication about me doing a shoot and interview for my fiftieth, but I didn't want to. I had stopped talking to the press. So it was over and out from me, and Matthieu suggested I put myself on the cover of *Frank* and do an interview. At first I thought it was a crazy suggestion; it would seem 'egotistical'. But he continued and asked, 'Why do you want to promote other people's magazines and not your own?' and with one excellent question he completely flipped my mind on it. I realised it was a fantastic opportunity. Finally, I could control how I wanted to look and, more importantly, what I wanted to say. So I arranged everything and conducted my own interview, and published it. I shot it with Elizabeth Hoff, a great photographer, and discussed the shots. The pictures were natural, strong, sexy and fresh – I was turning fifty, and it was exactly how I felt.

People had asked me what I would do for the big day for the whole year running up to it. My answer was always the same. 'I want to wake up with a man.' My friends thought it was hilarious, but I was just being honest. However, no man was in sight at those times, as I'd been single for ages, but right now I did have someone to ask.

I decided to go to Paris for a five-day break. I booked a stunning suite with a garden terrace and went for it. Matthieu was at a film festival in Rome, so I visited museums for the first three days and finally saw Monet's 'Water lilies' at The Orangery and the Rodin Museum; I sat in the Sacré-Coeur and said a little prayer. Things I hadn't done all those years ago.

I was worried that Matthieu might decide not to come. I had been let down so much by men that I had a nagging fear he might not show. But he did come, soon after landing from a film festival, and it was a relief to see him; I could relax and just hang out. He had arranged dinner at the Eiffel Tower, but all I wanted to do was chill in my beautiful suite and get room service. We did – and we had a brilliant night, and he was the best company.

The magazine was published the following day on my fiftieth birthday. Matthieu stayed for breakfast, took some birthday photographs of me, then went off into the heat of Paris, and I headed back to London for dinner with Adam and my friend Julie that evening and for the show with Alan the following day. Arriving at fifty was liberating. I felt like I had landed on a life raft where I had to stop giving a fuck what people said and continue to do what I bloody well wanted.

Chapter 18

Despite what was happening worldwide – with the challenging pandemic, the idle words used in government and loose-lipped contradictory information spewed, which I started to find irksome – 2020 was a pretty good year for me.

The wheels of the entertainment industry were grinding into action as everyone began to work out how to get back to production safely, and the shows I was involved with were actively looking for solutions. I was happy that my radio show and voice-over work could continue, and because the magazine was online I was able to keep it alive, too.

I hadn't left my flat in months, I'd been glued to the news and barely going out. So when the masks became mandatory, it was a godsend for me. Nobody recognised me for the first time in forever when I ventured out – unless I spoke, when my voice was a dead giveaway. So although I didn't particularly want to wear them, they worked in my favour. Travelling into the West End for my radio show and voiceover was strange. There were no people or cars anywhere. London was an eerie yet beautiful ghost town, and I loved the tranquillity of it all; without the sensory overload, I could tune into its beauty.

I bought myself a T-shirt that said: 'I love social distancing', which I put on Instagram. It upset a few people, but I did feel that way, and I still do. The energy of strangers had always been an issue for me. I realised I was highly empathetic, which dictated that I took on too much energy from others, and it took the pandemic to reveal how much all that had been affecting my mental health. Men always pulled me for a kiss on the cheek or had their hands around my waist. People being over-familiar with me when they had just met me made my skin crawl. I felt I couldn't show my discomfort or demonstrate my boundaries, and here we had the government enforcing distance, so I was happy. I now know these energy sensitivities are prevalent in autistic people, and that, coupled with high empathy, is exhausting.

Sarah Thomson-Woolley rang to tell me *The Great Pottery Throw Down* was recommissioned. The shoot would involve us being in a bubble at the pottery in Stoke-on-Trent for a few months. I had my radio show every Saturday in London, so no matter what, I had to be back for that. They had worked around those dates with lots of sorting and booking testing, so all we had to do was to agree on the money. The negotiation was in process.

I needed an amount that would help me do the job in the first place. The juggle over the summer holidays, the work, the boys, running my home, the energy it cost me – all the routine decisions you have to make around taking a job offer, and even though I loved the show, I knew my worth and told them what fee I required. I heard nothing.

I called Sarah a week later to ask if there was any news or wiggle room, but they had already offered the job to someone else. I couldn't believe it. Then when the production company was 'penning' their press release, they asked me if it was okay if they said it was for Covid reasons that I couldn't do the show. I said it was okay but later wondered why I hadn't encouraged them to tell the truth. We did not come to a financial agreement, and there is no shame in that. I still haven't watched the new shows. I'm sure they are utterly wonderful, but I can't bring myself to do it; I think because I know, despite my sensitivities, I could have gained confidence in the mechanics of the format and could have grown into the work and the role. My dad, having rarely really spoken to me about my work, mentioned to me recently that he thought it had been a good show for me, and he was right.

Show business holds a weird hierarchy where the channel is at the top, the production company is in the middle, and the talent is at the bottom. Agents tend not to play hardball in negotiations because they don't want to be seen as brutal and possibly lose work for other clients on their roster, so somehow you're supposed to feel lucky that you are in the mix for a job, a job that you are good at. And you are also made aware that you are easily replaced. It's a total headfuck.

I believe people bring their magic, unique gifts, a different charm, grace or skill set to the job, but treating it like a big stable is disrespectful and undermines all. All 'talent' have different needs, merits, levels of experience and lifestyles and should be treated as individuals. PR people also have to keep the press sweet so as not to jeopardise their relationships with them and perception of reliability. For example, I once had a call from my

PR agent because the press had got wind of something that happened between me and a famous man, which I perceived as nothing, so I denied it. I did not want it to be all over the press as I could predict it perpetuating the myths about me and the salacious nature of the 'reporting'. And since my eldest was in the middle of studying, I didn't want the story to jeopardise his concentration for the exams. More importantly, I wanted to maintain my privacy. So I told my PR to lie and say it wasn't remotely true. A year later, when they got wind of the 'lie', they printed it as if it was currently happening. I hadn't even seen him for over a year by that point – it was no longer 'news' – but they just went ahead and published it anyway. It was manipulative and vindictive, with no regard for its impact. My hatred of the press grew, and the system made me sick.

Determined to rise above it, I got back into working on my lovely magazine after all the lockdowns. The team and I were in Henley-on-Thames shooting a cover story, and I was in a giddy mood and enjoying the day. There was much talk about travel and where we all wanted to go. Europe had opened up again, and the one place I wanted to go was Venice.

I had only ever seen it in the movies and documentaries, and because of my love of art, architecture, water and beautiful things generally, I always knew I would love it. However, I had only ever imagined experiencing it with a perfect romantic partner. My fantasy was days spent with a handsome lover, meandering around the canals and bridges, eating good food and having lots of highly charged sex. I rang Matthieu to see if he would meet me there, but he was filming. While chatting to our hairdresser, Alex, on the shoot, he suggested I go alone, and I thought, why the hell not? I could be waiting my whole life for the right person to go with, or I could go and have the experi-ence right now for myself. One thing the pandemic had taught me was that life was too damn short. Then a friend and colleague piped up, 'I'll go with you,' which was unpredicted.

We got a great deal on a hotel the following week, booked early flights, and were on our way. It was a two-night delight, but I wouldn't have cared if I had been only there for two seconds after such a long time of wanting and waiting to go.

When we got on the water taxi, my eyes were on stalks, and I felt incredibly emotional. Seeing Venice on the horizon from the boat felt like a dream; I could not believe I was there. There were no crowds, due to Covid, and it felt like we had the city virtually to ourselves.

Our hotel was in the Dorsoduro district, which was perfect for me. Low-key, not so obvious, not touristy and laidback – absolutely my vibe. The sun was shining, and we dumped our bags in our rooms, went down to the hotel courtyard, ordered a bit of breakfast, and worked out what we would do for the rest of the day.

I was beside myself to get out there, and I drank it all in when we finally stepped out. Venice deeply moved me, and the call of the sailors and the sound of the water traffic were vibrant and nourishing for me. There was a hum of music in the air as church bells chimed along with the sounds of street music envelopes where visitors and locals collided; everyone just getting about their work, quests and adventures. Venice is alive, living on long deep breaths, and I was mirroring it and letting go.

We found a beautiful church selling tickets to watch a quintet playing Vivaldi's 'Four Seasons', so we booked tickets for the following night. Next, we strolled and found St Mark's Square; I could feel the history of it, revelled in the architecture and marvelled at how this beautiful city was constructed on the water. Finally, we ate lovely food, took in the sunshine, laughed, talked and immersed ourselves in the experience.

On Saturday morning, we got up and had breakfast. The weather was incredible again and we excitedly planned our day. As I ran upstairs to brush my teeth and organise my bag for leaving early the next day, I realised my passport was missing. I do lose things, it has to be said, but this felt odd. I looked everywhere; I was trying to breathe and not panic and was tearing around my room desperately, taking everything out of everywhere. I checked under the bed, in the drawers and in my toiletry bag. It was just gone, and I was in total panic. I ran back to my friend and told her the news, then I chatted with the concierge. The guy told us to report it to the police station, and we decided to retrace our steps from the previous day just in case we might find it. We had no joy.

So finally, the two of us sat in a cafe on St Mark's Square, me crying about how stupid I was, when we started to work out what I needed to do, which was to ring the Embassy, cancel the existing passport and apply for an emergency replacement, which would only be valid for my passage home. I squared it with Daniel that he was able to keep the boys until my return, whenever that was going to be, and convinced my friend to sort her life out so she too could stay for a couple more days to have some fun. After the initial panic and worry, to my joy, I realised I was stranded in Venice. The universe had well and truly taken over. It was crazy but also fate, and I was grinning from ear to ear.

We returned to the hotel, got everything organised, extended our stay and went out to have fun and do what we hadn't done on the first day, which was to go on a gondola ride.

It was my girlfriend who spotted him before I did. We were crossing the Accademia Bridge, and she started to do a little wolf whistle at the gondolier at the bottom of the stairs.

'Gondola ride, ladies?' he asked, and we looked at each other, laughed, and said yes, please.

He was utterly charming, kind, funny and very handsome. I noticed that he was clearing the rubbish from the canal and picking out plastic bottles as we went, and another gondolier was saying something aggressively in Italian. When I asked him what that meant, Riccardo told me he had said he shouldn't clean the canal when he had passengers in the boat. I told him I didn't mind and would do the same. I thought it was commendable that he loved his home and environment and, in my view, it was an admirable quality.

He told us about the history of Venice, and we relaxed back to enjoy the mellow ride. It was lovely to see the geography of the place from the water and the light and life buzzing everywhere. He flirted with me, then asked if we could 'go out and drink something'. I asked him how old he was, and he said it wasn't important. I liked his confidence a lot. When we were getting off the boat he asked me for my number, and now, with my newfound time in Venice ahead of me, I just thought fuck it, I like him, why not?

That night Vivaldi did not disappoint. My friend and I loved it, and as usual we ended up giggling at something ridiculous until we were silently laughing and tears were rolling down my face, as I desperately tried not to snort. However, the music was incredible, and it was a memorable evening. Riccardo messaged me and asked if I could meet him after the concert. I was too tired to see him, but I promised I would see him the next day.

We woke to a serious downpour, and Riccardo messaged to see if I was still up for meeting him. I agreed, but I needed to go out to get a few items of clothing first as I had only packed for two days. The rain was bouncing down now, and while my friend was up for hibernating in her room all afternoon, I was up for meeting Riccardo.

I told reception that I had a guest coming over and for them to see him to my room when he arrived. When I opened the door he was a sight for sore eyes, standing there looking stylish, out of his work uniform, immaculate and handsome. We just started talking, and I began to get my shoes on, ready to leave, when he just kissed me, and the chemistry was insane. He was intelligent, funny, respectful, and we were really into each other. For the rest of the trip, I was balancing my time getting to know him and having fun with my friend. She was over the moon for me and we had such a good time. Sadly, Riccardo and I were being photographed; I didn't know that some of our moments had been stolen. Then we started to see photographers every-where. It was a joke.

It was time for my friend to leave, so I said a tearful goodbye to her. The hotel informed me the lost passport had been found at the industrial laundry out of town. It had somehow got buried in my sheets. It had been on my bed all along. I was glad to get it back, but it was no longer valid, so I still had to wait for the emergency passport to arrive. So Riccardo took a day off work to spend with me.

He weaved through Venice, my hand in his. He was able to shake the paps with his impressive knowledge of the back streets and shortcuts of Venice. Finally, we escaped to the mainland to have a day together away from lenses and to get some privacy. After years of looking over my shoulder, he encouraged me to let go, and I needed it. He did not give a shit about my career, just me and who I was. We did not define the relationship in any way; we just went with the vibe, which was beautiful. He gave me faith again and opened my heart – not just in a romantic sense, but he reminded me that there are good people in the world who aren't out for what they can get, merely open to connecting. He also reminded me what it felt like to be cared about and looked after, not with words but with actions. It had been so long, indeed it may never have been. His energy matched mine; we were having so much fun, and I thought I had known him all my life. I'd never met someone so wise for their age, unguarded and open.

My visit to Venice held a spiritual awakening for me, as India had done before. I was healing further, and I felt well. I was starting to see more of the magic in my life and where it was happening; being open to experiences was the key to under-standing what the universe was showing me. I left Venice so sad to say goodbye, but knew I would see it and Riccardo again. It was pre-ordained, and it felt incredible.

The day after I left, some British journalist had hot-footed it to Venice, got into Riccardo's boat and tried to question him about me. When he rang to tell me, I was so upset. These disre-spectful wankers were on his beautiful boat, bothering this beautiful person. I was seething. Riccardo handled it well, but I told him to say 'no comment' if they asked anything more.

'Whatever you say, they can twist,' I told him. He preferred this approach and took my advice.

Having sat on the images for days, the press finally published them on Sunday. I knew they were waiting for the weekend, because they sell the most papers on Sunday. I pre-warned the boys and told them about my experience in Venice. Yet again, I had to tell my sons about my personal life before the papers splashed it everywhere in the sordid way they did, and before the gossip spread. Although my children would never judge me, no mother should be put in a position where she has to explain her romantic life to her children, no matter how old they are. But it was better they heard it from me over someone else's idle gossip.

One of the main reasons the press were all up in arms was that they reported Riccardo as being twenty-four (he was twenty-three), and I was fifty. I was a 'predator', which was the decades-long standard narrative for me, and he was a 'toyboy', which reduced this incredible human to nothing but a plaything. It was disrespectful to him and to me. It was disgusting.

Everyone was talking about us, even discussing us on TV and radio, and my direct messages on social media went mad. It triggered a varied response; primarily women celebrated me, which was interesting; while men sent me pervy messages. In the eyes of the press I had had a holiday 'fling', which meant that men assumed I might want to have a 'fling' with them, and many young men asked me out, thinking that their age alone would interest me.

The reality was that I was living my life; I had met someone who asked me out for a drink, and we liked each other. There was no fanfare or drama. I'd merely said yes. I found the assumptions, narrative and response bizarre. I was just being me.

Chapter 19

I was home, working and applying for a new passport, as I wanted to get back to Venice as soon as humanly possible. I had connected with the place, and it spoke to me. I had made some great contacts for interviews for the magazine, and journalists could travel, so I decided I would do some work on *Frank* and see Riccardo too.

I got all the paperwork and the letters I needed for entry, and as soon as my passport arrived I was gone. I called the team at ITN who were making the Des tribute show to tell them I was off to Italy and I'd be back to be able to do my master interview as soon as I returned. I was cutting it fine as they were finishing filming soon, but they said it was okay. I was dreading doing the interview because I always get emotional when speaking about Des, and I knew it would be hard. Des was not very well either and had been admitted to hospital, so I had been in touch with his daughter Kristina, and she was keeping me up to speed on how he was doing.

I arrived to serious Covid restrictions in Italy; masks still had to be worn outside, and curfew was 10.30pm. Where the streets previously had been quiet, they were now virtually empty. We unpacked in our rented apartment, popped out for take-out pizza before the restrictions came in, and went to bed.

I woke in the early hours to pop to the loo and checked my phone to see the time. I noticed I had a message from Kristina – saying that her father had died. I was beside myself. I didn't want to disturb Riccardo, so I got up, left the room and sobbed. I was trying to be quiet, but Riccardo woke and asked me what was happening. So I told him a dear friend had died and he held me as cried, until I fell asleep. I woke to that sad pit of loss in my belly. I explained to Riccardo who Des was and who he had been to me; he listened and supported me. In fact, he took care of me all day. I was a mess and grief-stricken.

I felt blessed that I was actually experiencing this with somebody to hold me, somebody to soothe me, and I was so happy not to be in the UK. My agent called to ask if I wanted to talk to anybody in the press. He was inundated with requests for me to appear on TV to speak about Des. My answer was no. I was grieving and couldn't speak anyway, and even if I could, I certainly wasn't going to talk to them. So instead I put a message on social media about my feelings for him, then backed off and dealt with it privately with the support of Riccardo.

I spent a lot of time thinking about Des. He always wanted to be positive, always looked on the bright side of life and always had a smile for me, and I acknowledged how much I appreciated him and loved him. I told him everything, and he had always championed me, never judged me and demonstrated only love. Filming for the documentary was still going, and I knew it would be even more emotionally charged now that he had died.

So I emailed production to square with them again about the date and if they could double check the rules and regulations around me coming home and quarantining. I thought I was okay because I had been working there, so they checked with the government guidelines and confirmed that that was correct and we could go ahead with filming on my return.

When I got home, I stayed in for two days before the filming. I didn't want to go anywhere, nor did I want to do the filming either. Then I arrived at the hotel suite for the recording, where it was all socially distant and a very small team. The guy interviewing me was on a laptop screen on a cushion raised for my eyeline, a first for me, and one other person who worked the sound and camera, then there was my make-up artist, Sally. It did not take long, it wasn't as bad as I thought it would be, and I didn't lose it.

I posted a picture of me outside of the hotel on Instagram. I was obligated to post a photo of a coat I had been gifted, and I knew that I would not have another chance to do it any time soon because I was not going to leave the house for a while. The next day a guy from the *Sun* was hounding my agent, desperate to run a story, hell-bent on painting me as a lawbreaker. I had, for the entire lockdown, stuck to the rules. 'What are they saying?' I asked. 'They want you to apologise for breaking lockdown rules.' I actually laughed, 'Apologise to the *Sun* newspaper? Ha! Over my dead body. What a fucking joke.' As far as I was concerned I had been in Italy legally, which is why I was let in, and I had stuck to government guidelines on my return.

I said nothing, and they ran the story with the pure intention of inciting hate towards me, which was completely unfair. I was hammered on social media by people who read this drivel and believed it. I was distraught. I had not done anything wrong, and the injustice stung deep.

After a day of abuse, I asked my agent to tell ITN to put out a statement to back me up, which they agreed to do. That night the boss of ITN rang me and said how upset everyone was, and told me his staff member who had checked the rules had been crying all day because of the 'mistake'. I reminded him that I also had been crying all day, and luckily for her, she could hide at the office and lick her wounds, but I was being dragged through the dirt publicly, and taking all the heat for it. I asked him to read me the statement, which he did. It did not cover me at all, it shoved me further under the bus, and I told him so. But he disagreed and said it would be fine.

The next day the statement, as predicted, buried me further, and I was seriously fed up. The press had whipped people up who were baying for my blood, leading one woman to message me to say, 'Even ITN have washed their hands of you.' I was furious, so I decided to take matters into my own hands. I'm a fifty-year-old woman and I'm still letting these bastards bully me, so I thought, fuck it, if no one defends me, I will defend myself. So I redacted the names and email addresses and published the emails from the production team on my Instagram account. My email asked if it was okay by the rules that I do the interview after my return to England, and the producer checked and responded, yes.

The first message that came up on my feed was from a mate just saying 'Mic drop,' and that's precisely what it was. All the trolling I had suffered over the last forty-eight hours stopped and the news story disappeared. It was quashed immediately. I was sick and tired of having my reputation wiped across the floor. I woke up to my agent calling me: ITN had been ringing, and what should he say? I simply said, 'Get them to call me.' It was no surprise to me when they never did.

I ended up not leaving my house for the next sixteen days. I never wanted to go out anyway, and even less now. I didn't want to see anyone; I was devasted, still grieving Des, juggling everything alone as always, and I could not believe how I was continuing to be treated. My personal trainer messaged me and said you've got to get out; the gym is empty, please come. So I got my shit together and started the short walk to meet him. As soon as I walked out of the door I heard the buzz of a car window going down, and as I looked up I saw the huge lens and heard the clicks of the camera. A man was just shooting me in a car outside my flat. I walked straight over to him, and he put the camera down. 'What are you doing here?' I said. 'People are just interested in you,' he told me. 'But this is my home,' I said. 'Do you want me to leave?' he asked. 'Yes, please,' I answered, and he drove off.

I have no idea how many days that man had camped out there waiting for me to break 'isolation', waiting for another news story. I had no freedom in this country and was increasingly happy staying indoors. I just didn't understand why all this was happening; I was being drawn into this drama and stalked left, right and centre. All I wanted to do was live my life in peace.

I was quite depressed as Des's funeral approached. It was a small affair with all the Covid funeral restrictions, and I had received the details at the last minute like everyone else, so the press would not get wind of it. I decided to listen to one of Des's albums in the morning. Every time he sang, I was, without fail, moved to tears; such is the kindness that comes from it. I knew I had to get some tears out of my system before I got to church. It was a massive release and I'm glad I did it. It helped a lot. Everyone had to social distance, and I arrived and sat alone. It wasn't easy, but it was an honour to be there and say goodbye to my wonderful friend.

The rest of 2020 was pretty grim; I was crushed and had darkness in my heart. Riccardo was struggling to come over to London, and the lockdowns complicated everything, so I pulled the plug on it.

After that, Christmas was just a complete no-go zone; it was always a difficult time for me and would induce depression annually. Daniel had agreed at the beginning of our separation that the kids could always wake up with me on Christmas morning, no matter what. And we alternated Christmas dinners and Boxing Day each year. Of course, I loved it just being the three of us, but I was always mindful that the kids might prefer the extended family experience. Roman liked the balance of both, and Valentino preferred to be quiet like me; he's always happy where I am. So this year, when they left for their dad's, I was down but managed to make a full Christmas dinner for one and got ready for a day of watching films and enjoying the peace. I had asked for David Lean's *Summertime* as a Christmas present, which was a film my friend Russell Norman had encouraged me to see because of my Venice story. He thought it might resonate. I thought I'd seen all of Lean's movies, so it was a delightful surprise to find I'd been missing this one. Katharine Hepburn and Venice were incredible, and the storyline was compelling. I can always lose myself in a film.

A month or so before the Christmas break I had been asked if I would like to do *Celebrity MasterChef*. I absolutely loved to cook and I had hosted a cooking show before, so I had insight into how it was done. I had also had a great experience on *Bake Off* and fronted a similar style of show with *The Great Pottery Throw Down*, so I thought I had a good sense of it, and it would be safe to agree to. I hoped that I might learn something, but more than anything I wanted to meet new people and have fun. But I made a huge schoolgirl error; I hadn't watched the show for over a decade, so in reality I had no idea what I was really letting myself in for.

There is a big build-up to the show and lots of preparation. Production is nurturing and keeps you prepped as to what will happen and what you need, and I felt like I was entering a good show. So on the first day of filming, the first question that Gregg Wallace, one of the presenters, asked out of all the millions of questions he could have opened with, was, 'So, models, do they eat?'

I was shocked. I'm standing in front of all the cameras with twenty-five years' worth of broadcasting experience under my belt; I've been in his shoes a million times, and this is how he introduces himself to me and me to the show? It was a poor combination of zero homework, assumption, ignorance and disrespect with an extra helping of arrogance. He could not interview his way out of a paper bag, and, needless to say, when the show was aired his opener hit the cutting-room floor. I was not impressed in the slightest. My back was well and truly up as he tried to hold court and peacock around.

The drill was that we cooked something, and the judges would then ridicule us for what we thought we knew and shame us for the things we didn't, so that they had options for the edit and a nice head-fuck for us. My confidence deteriorated by the day.

At the same time, I was continuing filming for *Shop Well for Less* and another show, *Shop Well for the Planet*. I was tired, swamped and not enjoying any of the work. I had slowly been sucked back in again, and nothing had changed. I had completely and utterly outgrown television and how it was made.

The *MasterChef* experience continued to be an eye-opener, and some unprofessional behaviour on set was jaw-dropping. I was in a cycle of desperately wanting to leave but also wanting to do well because I was in a competition. One of the challenges was to make a monstrous sandwich; I could not believe I was on *MasterChef* learning how to make a fucking sandwich. This challenge was a crime against focaccia. I just could not do it. So I decided to make a small chicken ciabatta sandwich because I did not give two hoots at this point. I had not stuck to the brief, but no one asked why. It was bizarre. I asked if I could have it for lunch after they had filmed it. It was delicious.

I kept getting through the rounds, and I started to ask if the other contestants were actually enjoying it, because I wasn't, and slowly people began to air the things that had happened to them. But they were just dealing with it, like I was trying to.

I've always been really professional; at work I am always present and have a discipline that I am proud of. I always do my homework. And despite Gregg barking orders behind the scenes about how we had to behave, I found him very unprofessional. I hate injustice and double standards, and I could see the presenters were at a loss to help anyone. When I was finally out, I wanted to run out of there, I could not wait to leave, but I did try to find John to say goodbye; he had obviously wanted to get out of there as much as I did, as he had already left.

As I was walking to the car, Gregg was leaving too, and he said, 'Appearing on this will do a lot for you.' I didn't know what to say, so I smiled and said yes, but I was really thinking, 'Yes, you have finally helped me decide to end my television career once and for all.' I was done.

A colleague suggested that we both focus on the magazine more now that I had more time to make it into a business, and that we should really make a go of it and turn it into a website. I was only too happy to do so, it was a welcome break from TV and we were full of new ideas for its direction.

Between friends introducing me to some ethical brands and my work on *Shop Well for the Planet*, my eyes had been opened to the climate crisis. I was focused on how as individuals we could change our habits to not compound the problem but to help slow down and eventually put the brakes on it killing us. Until that point, I'd heard of carbon footprint but I hadn't fully understood what it meant.

I also wanted to support and celebrate the women doing amazing things in the world, and interview them in their chosen fields and ventures. Instead of continuing with the over-forty focus, I decided to open up the magazine to women of all ages. After the news of what happened to Sarah Everard at the hands of a policeman that March, women's safety was a huge topic in the media, and it was clear that the threat was literally everywhere, even among the people employed to protect us. It resonated so strongly with me, and I was sickened and devastated by her tragic experience. I chatted with my circle of female friends and women at work and it seemed everyone had a story about some man behaving threateningly or inappropriately. It was insane. Things surfaced that women had minimised, including me, for fear of not being believed or because we have been simply programmed to not really see it as wrong, with the everyday sexism we endured embedded in our psyche as normal and acceptable.

I wanted to shake things up and start using my magazine as my voice, where my words could not get twisted and might even help some people. It was a new vibe, and we had three months to work hard on the content ready for the big relaunch. I was excited, motivated and pumped for the future.

Chapter 20

In the early months of the pandemic, an extremely close friend asked me if I would like to invest in her new business. It was a project that I thought might help many people, but I am not a gambler. Even when I was little, if Mum gave us 50p to go on the slot machines on holiday, I would always keep my winnings because walking out of the arcade empty-handed didn't feel good. So I told her I wasn't interested but wished her well with her venture.

Over the next few days and weeks, she assured me it would be risk-free, and she promised me that she would do me a special deal where whatever I put in, I would get back with or without the interest. She told me her family were also investing because it was that much of a dead cert, and I'd met her family, and they were lovely, hard-working people, and I honestly thought if they were doing it, it must be safe. I went for it. I handed over my savings and tax savings as I had time to get the money back and pay my tax bill. I forgot about it and got on with work.

I was working on the *Shop Well* format; its intentions were good, and all the sharing of doable tips to help people get Earth-friendly was important. It helped me reconnect with my father's influence – his voice in the 1970s and his activism around environmental issues. I felt very proud of him and became dedicated to making change in my life, becoming mindful of the Earth, wherever and whenever possible. As a result, I stopped buying new clothes, shopping instead only from charity and thrift shops; I was determined not to add to the ever-growing landfill that was literally choking our world. I changed what I used in the house and became conscious of everything I bought, asking myself, where did it come from? Where was it going once I'd finished with it?

I was avoiding plastic like the plague and trying to educate the boys on how to live more sustainably. I unfollowed people on social media who weren't really adding anything to my life and started to align with the like-minded. I looked for more ethical accounts that cared about the environment so I could get an education. I was exploring the movement and couldn't believe how asleep I'd been. I was on a mission, learning and reading a lot, which made me feel good. Other people around me were also very much part of that change, showing me things of interest or putting me on to people who could help us so I could connect with them and expand what we were doing.

This meaningful pursuit cast a light on the nonsense that went with filming TV shows – even ones with eco-friendly messages. Nothing about them rang true – often despite environmental messaging in the programme, productions weren't practising what they preached. Plastic water bottles and plastic-covered catering were on set every day. It reminded me that in telly it's not about what is being said, it's about how it appears. It is, after all, called a 'show'. This was the exact opposite of what I believed; I realised that this was one of the causes of the internal friction I had felt all these years.

Nevertheless, I loved meeting new people and as always, helping the contributors, as they are known – the people who we were focusing on who were not from television but appearing on screen for the first time. They were great and fun to befriend, and I enjoyed making them feel at ease on shows like *Shop Well*, supporting them, and ensuring they had a positive experience.

Alongside juggling filming days and the magazine, it was time for me to get my money back from the investment, but my friend kept telling me it was coming, then telling me why it wasn't coming yet. I now had seriously diminishing funds; I was about to retire from TV and had invested in my magazine. This was not a time for lies; I needed that money back. It was my hard-earned cash. It belonged to the tax man and me.

I was getting increasingly stressed and alarmed. This person had seen everything about me through my darkest times. Finally, I began to get tired of her out-and-out lies and persistent fobbing off, so a close colleague told me I should file it with the police and get a lawyer. So I did.

I couldn't believe it. My friend of six years had scammed me. I was brokenhearted. What niggled me the most was that I had all the signs that this person was a liar, but I had ignored them. Her stories were becoming wilder, and I had been warned early on that she wasn't what or who she said she was. But unfortunately I did not fully tune into the message and ignored the alarm bells.

I was also at the end of my TV career and only survived those last few shows with the help of Sally, my make-up artist, and Joanna's support. I just could not get past the charade, though, of not having told my colleagues about my plans, and on the last day of filming, just before my final setup, I told Joanna I was retiring. She gave me a huge hug before we heard action and had to step out, and I had to remember my bloody lines one last time. In the car home, I felt waves of relief. Never would I put myself in that position again.

On the magazine, my friend and I were working brilliantly together and had such fun as well. I felt happy that she was in my life. We were back and forth to Venice, avoiding social media to be free, have fun, and make connections. It was incredible.

We flew again to Venice for my fifty-first birthday to celebrate and get more work done on *Frank*, and the months since my retirement from telly felt terrific. However, in the run-up to the magazine launch I started to feel that something wasn't quite right. My friend wasn't sharing the website yet, and I was getting worried. I had asked her a few times if I could see it, but she was not forthcoming and I started to feel uneasy, but I pushed the feelings aside. She wouldn't lie to me, I thought, she knows everything I've been through. She also knew the depth of incision from my latest betrayal and she assured me everything was in hand for the launch. So, of course, I believed her.

My creative juices were flowing, and opportunities were coming to the fore. I got a call from someone at the BBC who wondered if I'd be interested in doing a documentary about autism and education. She had once been one of my producers during *The Big Breakfast* days. I told her I was out of the business, but I was contemplating making documentaries myself. I told her I would only get involved if I had complete control; if so, I might be interested. So she said that that wouldn't be a problem and I could call her sister about it as she too had children who were autistic, and she wanted me to talk about the inadequacies of the education system in terms of provision for autistic children. She had already spoken to an autistic advocate, and she asked me if I would be interested in talking to him. I contacted him and arranged a video meeting.

Creating the magazine platform was a full-time job; I was at my desk for all hours of the day and night and doing way too much for one person. I was wearing every hat imaginable. I was writing, editing and doing interviews, establishing contact with PR companies and trying to secure advertising, to name a few roles. There were people out there whose entire job was just one of these roles, and I was juggling all of them.

My first deal was with Scott at Phox Water, who was brilliant and fun to do business with. I had changed over my water filter during my conversion to a more eco-friendly life, and his product was one of the first swaps I made. So I just contacted him to start working out a deal with the magazine and me. It was beautiful, and I was looking forward to more transactions like that. Each of these successes was individually enjoyable, but collectively it wasn't easy. My friend and colleague was supposed to be doing her side of things, and every time I had a problem she told me not to worry; she could deal with it.

I was going through a very fertile period creatively, educating myself on the issues in the world and exploring documentaries on climate change and natural medicines, as well as the riches of the Earth and social structures. I watched documentaries like *Seaspiracy*, *The Minimalists* and *Weed the People* on Netflix, which broadened my mind. I was distilling the information I needed and making connections around these topics. And I was inspired to start helping to make a change. I wanted to make my own documentaries and was finding inspiration everywhere, so I began writing a list of films I wanted to make – such as about the fashion industry versus the planet, about medical cannabis – and I had an ever-growing list of ideas.

A friend introduced me to Dr Callie Seaman, a cannabis scientist and activist for change around these natural medicines. The 'weed' documentary was about how cannabis helps treat cancer, and here I was hearing about the many poorly children with epilepsy in the UK, and who, with the help of cannabis, were experiencing fewer seizures. It was a critical component in changing the quality of their lives and that of their carers. I met with Matt Hughes, the founder and director of MedCan Support, and Hannah Deacon, the woman who was instrumental in changing the legislation in the UK around getting access to prescriptions for cannabis on the NHS. They are a brilliant bunch of people, and my head was further blown; I wanted to help get the word out there, so I became their ambassador.

I needed someone with experience to work on the magazine and was advised to invest in a features editor, which I did in the form of the wonderful Victoria Earle, a lovely, talented person with a gorgeous heart who believed in what I was doing.

I called a meeting at my flat to prepare for the launch of *Frank*. The team gathered all the articles together so we could see what we had and what still needed doing. We were meant to be shown the website but instead my friend handed us pictures of it. She was behaving strangely – still we had not seen the site and we were due to launch in days. So after pressing her about what was going on, it became apparent that she had subcontracted out the building of the website to someone else, someone I didn't even know existed, and that it was nowhere near ready.

I was starting to do little videos here and there and on Instagram. I was sharing small updates on what was happening with the magazine and the problems with the launch. I talked about what was moving me then and how I felt they were well received. I had told myself over the years that I couldn't do this talking-to-camera thing, and putting videos on Instagram horrified me, so I set up a practice run and ended up broadcasting it. I realised I could be more me when I was alone and unwatched. I learned that the lens wasn't the problem but having people behind it – onlookers, production, just people.

I was always self-conscious about an audience, so my ability to do this freely was a surprise to me. People really liked it, so I started doing more of it. I realised I was helping people as I had always done in real life, and now I could do it for many more. I had always enjoyed motivating people, allowing them to see how I see them, and now I could do it for a bigger reach. It was such a good feeling. I've always been good at troubleshooting; I am solution-driven, not wanting to focus on a problem but on a route out of it. Through this, I got down to several of my issues, asking difficult questions and breaking things down. I have always tried to help people come out from behind their excuses, live more authentically, and make changes. So my energy was getting out there in my authentic voice direct from my heart and soul. I was visualising a *Frank* podcast and how to shoot some video content for the magazine and how it could grow.

However, I couldn't get too excited about the magazine because things were not good. I finally got an email from my friend saying she was distraught because she had no idea how to build a website, and had not known how to tell me; instead, she had chosen to lie to me for months. Nevertheless, a website with months of hard graft ready to publish and paid sponsors helping us get off the ground had only just started to be built.

It was the most bizarre scenario I had ever found myself in, because at what point did she think that she wouldn't get found out? This lie had a deadline that was the exact deadline of the magazine publishing day. She well and truly shafted me and pushed me further into debt.

I couldn't breathe, and to add insult to injury she tried to get legal with me, which hurt further. It was hit after hit. She slowly handed over the project, and I was in constant contact with the web designer. I ploughed in money, getting the help of someone who promised to turn this mess around, but she failed and I paid her anyway. I hate having debts but I was in the middle of a crisis, so instead I did what I could to keep things moving even though I was financially down even further. And then I got locked out of the site.

This was my second female hit the same year, and my spirit started to die. I could feel it. I'd given up the career that was hurting me and gone straight into being burnt by individuals. I threw myself into my new life without knowing that people could shaft me. I felt so stupid and low. How could I keep inviting this into my life? I know people are flawed, but through my lens I only see the good in people and their potential even when they cannot see it themselves. So I tap into that and how I can help, I believe what they tell me, ignore the warnings without any regard for myself and go even further to emotionally hold them. I am a sitting duck for narcissists and the perfect bait for people who take advantage.

Realising that I had been demonstrating this behaviour with men was bad enough – my second marriage was the big wake-up call, but the realisation that this has also been happening with women cut me deep. It hurt more than any injustice from men. Friends who had been privy to all my tears and witnessed my devastation in many situations could still hurt me. My heart had been broken again, and my ability to financially support my children was in danger. I was on my knees and every bit of money that was to come in would have to go on legal fees. I was not just in fear of losing my website, but losing everything.

I told a friend about what had happened, and she offered to help and sent me some money to alleviate the pressure. I hated debt and owing people money, but I needed help. I had explored the idea that Daniel would take the boys while I sold things and tried to reshape my life, but for now that could be held off.

Despite this, I felt I had to park my disappointment and keep moving forward and keep my magazine and my new business alive. My ex-brother-in-law, Simon, is a lawyer and he reconnected with me regarding me doing some charity work, so we went for lunch. We had not seen each other for years, and it was so good to catch up, as he was just a kid the last time I saw him. I told him about my situation with the investment, and he said he would like to represent my case, so when the shit went down with the magazine he put me in touch with a businesswoman, who could salvage the wreckage and help me reclaim ownership of the magazine and the name. It was an awful wait.

These were my new lessons in business, and they were huge. First, she helped me reboot the whole situation. She taught me things about the site; she refreshed me on how to do WordPress if I needed it and took a deeper look at the site in detail. Rebooting the entire site helped me understand WordPress again and showed me how to post so that I understood what was happening behind the scenes. I was steaming ahead, but inside I was falling apart. So I flew to Venice to be with Riccardo, and he helped me by just being there for me. I walked and walked and went to the gym, cooked food for us and worked.

While I was there, I had a Zoom meeting with a technical advisor about the autism documentary. He was articulate and intelligent, and we got on well. We arranged for him to come over to mine when I returned from Italy to talk further about the documentary and get to know each other. I relaunched the magazine without fanfare and I started work with Simon to get my savings back. Everything from now on would have to go on survival and legal bills.

I'd taken on a lot; I no longer had an agent, and any enquiries about work were now coming directly to me. I was fielding all this stuff and I was overloaded – it was a lot to handle. My rent was getting too high, too, and I was struggling to pay it, so I asked my landlord if she could hold my rent for a few months and that I would give it all back then, which she agreed to do, and I did. I sold my car and jewellery and some watches I had. I downsized my entire life financially. I was drowning in paper-work and I knew I had to ask for help but I didnt know where to turn.

I was using meditation as always to alleviate my stress, and during one session Shaima's name came to me. Shaima was a wonderful woman who worked at my local gym. She also did PR for charities and occasionally wrote articles for *Frank*. She had also been there for me when I decided to try a new gym class a few months back and the experience turned sour. It was a martial arts class, and my coordination was all out of whack, as it tends to be, there was not much room and my legs are long and were everywhere they shouldn't be. In addition, a lady next to me kept getting angry and giving me horrible looks. I explained that I was new, but she would not leave me alone. Her huffing and puffing and glaring at me really unravelled me, and I ended up leaving the class prematurely in tears. My coordination can be awful, but that woman had been so unkind. I reported the incident to Shaima, who was supportive and said she would sort it out.

Shaima was brilliant, kind and a hard worker, so I reached out to her and she came over immediately. I was a mess, and not only had I been entirely shafted by friends, but I was exhausted and needed help, and she slowly helped me through the tsunami of shit I was drowning in. We talked about her life, and I talked about mine and all that I've been through, and we broke everything down into bite-sized chunks, and things started to seem a little more manageable.

One day we were talking about how people perceive me, and she told me that the woman who had been mean to me in the gym all those months ago had gone to reception and complained that she did not want a 'husband beater' in her class. How could anyone seriously think me violent? I thought it was extraordinary, and although it was hard to hear I needed to listen to it.

If you looked me up online, it was all there, the twisted story, but the revocation of the caution was hardly reported, only getting a postage-stamp-sized piece in a tabloid on the day I received it. We talked about how I had never publicly discussed what had happened that night, and yet I had seen and been reading about how that night's experience was not uncommon, that women often get taken away in a domestic situation, and I was staggered. Shaima asked me why I'd never spoken to the press about my side of the story, and I explained that protecting the boys from situations like that is always at the heart of my reasoning.

At first I was adamant I would never speak to the press, but I did want to speak out. I wanted to talk about what was happening with the police and the ugly truth of their misogyny. How innocent women were being taken away and children were left with the perpetrator. I wanted to talk about these arrests of women where the police seem convinced by the gaslighting man.

I also needed to eliminate some of the trauma that had dogged my life over the years. Ever since the arrest I had been travelling and meeting new people to try to feel like a human being, and I knew people would google me and that story just would be there. So I had to tell new acquaintances that if they looked me up, stuff about me on there was not true. Literally all of it. It was demeaning. Over the years I had convinced myself that by never speaking of it I was somehow rising above it, and that I was protecting the boys, but I was kidding myself. It hadn't worked, and I needed to release the truth. The children were older now, so Shaima encouraged me to do an interview with *The Times* to get the message out there.

Meanwhile, the autism documentary was starting to take shape. My advisor and I eventually met in the flesh, and he came over. We could now create a document about what kind of film we wanted to make and prepare a programme treatment. So I made some lunch, and we talked. Then while we were hatching a plan he observed me and suggested I demonstrated ADHD behaviours. He suggested it might be good to get assessed and maybe try to get a test to see if I was autistic too. It was incredible to hear this, it had never been said to me before, and I was intrigued. It wasn't a shock, and I can even go as far as to say I knew he was right, and I was excited at the prospect of being diagnosed.

I started to explore my character; it was like a Rolodex of moments, feelings and thoughts – how I always just kept going, how I was always making notes, all the time being productive. I did drive myself nuts and would often sit myself down and say out loud, 'For fuck's sake, Melanie, can you just stop?' I felt like I was going crazy some days. One mission after another, one passion, one hobby after another, searching for information. I was going over and over scenarios in my head – good and bad ones – like a broken record; I now know it is a condition called echolalia, which is a common co-existing condition with autism. I was pursuing the truth in a world that does not care for it, and my foresight felt like torture, seeing every outcome and scenario, yet everyone else seemed blind to it.

I was still practising meditation and yoga at home but I wasn't feeling any lasting calm. I have always felt different to everyone I meet, and I see things differently, but I didn't know why, so with all the deep breathing in the world I didn't understand who I was, and with these few words my life immediately started to make sense and I could see how this knowledge might just unlock all the answers to my questions. I began to see myself for the first time. The more I explored, the more I came up trumps.

But we had work to do. We had to crack on, thrash around ideas and get down the story for the documentary. What did we want to say? What did we want to find out? What were we trying to teach people? Those types of questions. We knew it was about the education system and challenging it to find out why it was set up the way it was in the first place. It crushes creativity and individuality out of people, for any child, let alone autistic ones. It is a system that is failing most neurodivergent people and we had to think how we could shed light on what and how it is failing and how we could change it. We gave it a title, gave it a reason and just wrote down some of our thoughts about who we wished to interview and how we would stop this issue.

We finished our meeting excited about what we were going to do next. I immediately applied privately for an assessment for autism and ADHD – it would sink me further into debt, but I needed to do it for clarity. First, it would be the autism assessment in the following months, then I had to wait three months for the ADHD one. It finally arrived after three days of examinations via Zoom, which consisted of questions, tests and conversations. Now I just had to wait for the result.

I was in a meeting when the email came through, which confirmed that I indeed was autistic. I had to read it a few times to make sure I wasn't getting it wrong. First, I had to let myself believe what I was reading, then I looked up and told my colleague, 'I've just been diagnosed autistic.' I was over the moon – I finally had an answer.

I went to tell Ligita, too. I was overcome with gratitude. I had had fifty-one years to get through, and the process felt good, but I knew it would get more challenging. I told my boys and my mum and dad, and the following morning I put a video on Instagram to tell everyone my news, which was picked up by the press very quickly. I was inundated with requests to be interviewed about it, so I said yes to one radio show, *Woman's Hour*, which I thought would be an intelligent conversation, one TV show, *Loose Women*, because my friend Penny was going to be on there, one magazine, *Hello*, because they don't mess with what you say too much, and one newspaper, *The Times*, for similar reasons.

Shaima helped orchestrate it, and I organised the shoots and everything. Every production company wanted me to now do a documentary about the late diagnosis. However, I still wanted to tackle the education system as a broader subject. I did not like how the mainstream media made crap shows about autism with so-called experts who aren't even neurodivergent and always talk to autism awareness charities that are mostly run by neurotypicals. It, in my view, is total bollocks. So I did not go with anyone. I would have to do it my way, and I still had a lot of homework to do.

On top of that, I needed a therapist. I needed help to get me through this new information, this new autistic lens on my life and what it was showing me. So he put me on to the most brilliant woman, who is autistic herself and late diagnosed. She understands the autistic experience, and talking to her was an eye-opener and a heart-opener. I was unearthing lots of my life trauma. We discussed all my sensitivity, self-medicating, wide-open empathy levels, and how much I had blocked out, trying to pinpoint the moment I had started to mask. Morphing myself into whatever others deemed appropriate within the family and later relationships, work and society at large.

The therapist gave me lots of literature about trauma. She warned me to go easy. It was tough going, and it was Christmas, not my favourite part of the year, so it was very shaky ground for me, and the book cracked me open even more. All the denial of my life and all that I put up with started to come out. The book was tapping into my pain, and I became very depressed, but it was only because I was doing the work. I was going back to the beginning and digging into the hurts. Trying to remember who I was. I started to listen to the music of my youth to stimulate old feelings in my teenage years.

I just had to get through the Christmas period. I had a lovely morning on Christmas Day with the boys and held myself together, but I collapsed in a heap when they left. During the day I was curled up in a ball on the floor. I was howling like a wounded animal, and all my pain was coming out. I realised how much I had been running and running. And here I was, just a heap of exhausted flesh and bones with a crushed spirit. I started to wonder what it had all been about and what had been the point. I even explored the idea of why I should go on, what was the point? The answer was always 'for my boys'. It was my boys, unbeknownst to them, who had always been my saviours.

Chapter 21

I picked myself off the floor and had the Christmas lunch of my choice: a packet of chicken noodles and a small cheeseboard. Then I watched BAFTA screeners movies and cried and cried. I felt very alone and desperate. The depression felt primal, more profound than anything that had come before. My core wounds were entirely exposed, and I did not know how to soothe them.

I was in the process of being a judge for two large book prizes, so I had loads of books to read over Christmas and New Year, and I was heavily into watching my BAFTA screeners ready for voting, too, so at least my mind was preoccupied. These commitments held me together in one way, but I was aching for a break.

I was agoraphobic in London due to the press. They had been on my case all the time. I had no desire to leave and was always worried about being followed and papped. I was incarcerated in my home and had no incentive to go out, so I needed desperately to get out of London. I needed to be by the water and see some vast skies.

Luckily, I'd been offered a stay at a stunning coastal hotel in Cornwall for some PR on social media. I was also in possession of a hybrid Lexus that had been loaned to me in exchange for a piece in my magazine. It had been sitting outside unused for weeks, so I asked Riccardo if he fancied coming over to go to Cornwall, to show him a different part of England and share the driving, and so I could get familiar with the car. He said yes.

I finally managed to catch up with my sister Samantha before I left. I told her everything. She told me to keep in touch with her and we would speak more when I got back. I was relieved to be connected with her again.

Riccardo arrived; we had a few days in London before we left, which mostly I did not like. I was pushing myself so that Riccardo could have a nice time. I was stuck in a groove of wanting to ensure he was okay by doing what he wanted to do instead of taking care of me. Optimistically, I thought I could push my boundaries with him because I trusted him, and I felt safe when he was near. But the truth was that everything was daunting. Riccardo struggled to understand what had happened to me and why I had changed. They were dark rainy days, but we did have some fun. I took him to Cliveden, my favourite hotel in England, for lunch and a trip on the Thames. We also went to Camden, somewhere I hadn't been to for a while. We stumbled across an indoor golf place and he encouraged me to go and have a round. Unbeknownst to me, maths never being my strong suit, I won by ten points, and it did not go down very well and revealed a lot about Riccardo. I warned him if he didn't like this win then he should never go shooting with me.

We looked around the Tate Modern and crossed the

Millennium Bridge. The rain was driving sideways, and the sky was low and grey. We huddled under an umbrella and walked past a homeless guy who had recognised my voice a few minutes later and called to me. 'Hello Melanie,' he said, and told me how much he used to enjoy *Des and Mel* and how happy he was to see me. I threw him a smile and waved. I pondered his journey to where he was and how grateful I was to him for making me feel good about my old show. I only want to lift people's spirits; it's the thing I love doing the most.

Seeing how my emotions were wrapped up in my sensitivities was interesting. The Tube was overwhelming; the noise, the people, the tannoy and the levels of sounds affected my hearing; I couldn't talk or fight above it. And I had no desire to. I had to take deep breaths. We still had to use our masks on public transport, so I didn't fear being recognised; otherwise I would not have been there. Finally, after enduring the assaults of London for a few days, I was more than ready to get my arse down to Cornwall.

We arrived, and the hotel was lovely and the view beautiful. The weather was glorious, and I wanted to sit outside to eat. I did not want to be inside on this treasure of a January day, but Riccardo did. I needed to be out, which rankled him and, in the process, rankled me. I was feeling irritable, angry and on edge.

After lunch, we returned to the room and Riccardo asked, 'Are you okay, because you don't seem it?' 'No, I'm not,' I said and started crying. I felt something rupture, like the illusion of me shattered, and my tears turned to convulsions that felt violent and frightening. The room was spinning, and I had to lie down. I was shaking and nauseous. Riccardo came to hold me and the tears flowed. Realising that I had been living on my last nerve for years was hard to bear. In all these years I was never in flow with myself, constantly battling against the tide, and now it all gave way to cries of pain that were sonorous and wretched.

I knew it was a nervous breakdown. I was in it, thinking, 'My God, this is what people mean when they talk of nervous breakdowns. This is it.' I couldn't get my breath, so Riccardo took control. He put his nose to mine and asked me to follow his breathing to regulate my own so I didn't hyperventilate. He brought me to a calmer state and eventually, miraculously, I was relaxed enough to sleep. He was just incredible.

When I woke, I had no strength in my body – all those years of holding on, I had released. I had been fighting to survive, running at and through my problems, never giving myself time to heal and lick my wounds. I finally realised that all my demons, mistakes and shameful things that I had thought I had to hide and all my darkness had stepped forward. I knew it was a monumental moment, a huge turning point. I had finally caught up with myself, and it had not been pretty. It was now 'do or die'.

I rose the next day to get myself together for a long Zoom meeting. I had to help choose the winner of one of the book prizes. So I zipped myself up, got my shit together one last time, and appeared to the panel as if nothing had happened. I would get this done and dusted then focus on my recovery, get out in Cornwall and try to relax with Riccardo.

We talked about what had happened, and he said he'd found it easy to help me, but he had been quite scared for me. I will be forever grateful for his strength. We had four more days to walk, talk and visit the beaches. I occasionally laughed amongst oceans of tears, and Riccardo rolled with it and supported me.

Introducing a Venetian to a cream tea was hilarious: he could not understand the use of all the fat and sugar. It offended his palate, which made me laugh a lot, and when a bloody big seagull descended on him and tried to steal his crepe I thought I was going to pee myself laughing.

We visited a tired-looking arcade to play the slots and other delights. I settled on the shooting range while Riccardo explored. When I caught up with him, he was on a game where he was throwing an endless supply of balls at what appeared to be a row of bottles in a vending machine. Every time he hit one, it made the satisfying sound of shattering glass, which I hadn't realised was a sound I exquisitely enjoyed. He insisted I have a go. 'It will be good for you.' Once I started, I was like a whirling dervish, in a frenzy of letting out loads of pent-up anger and getting my heart rate up. I loved it. Riccardo is always so good at understanding what I need and getting me to do things out of my comfort zone, knowing what would benefit me. Well, he gets it right most of the time.

We saw some sunsets that were good for the soul, and I tried to keep my head down and not be recognised, but unfortunately a few people were trying to take pics of me from a distance. Over the years, people have been attempting to steal images of me wherever I go. Whenever I moaned to a friend about being a known face and recognised, I minimised my pain by caveating it with 'I know I'm not (insert any globally known person here)', but the intrusion was permanent, and I hated it. I'd rather someone say hi and exchange words than take a snap of me surreptitiously. I hate how it feels. The most obvious is when people pretend to be doing a selfie where I am in the back of the shot. It's a technique I have seen used by people on the escalators or in queues if I am behind them. Once people clock me, I watch them, but they don't notice me observing them, as if somehow I am deaf or blind. The truth is that all of my senses are well and truly on, and if I were to ask them to stop, somehow I would be painted as a bitch, the 'Who does she think she is?' syndrome.

I don't think of myself as 'anyone'; I am just me. If you are trying to get a picture, ask yourself why you want a picture of me or anyone for that matter. Do you think I am someone, and why? My job was my job, not a route to fame.

We made our way back to London, then Riccardo had to leave; I realised I needed to listen to myself, take time out for the first time in my life and stop everything. No quick fixes; this situation in my life had to be handled carefully and respectfully. That situation being me.

I called my GP to ensure my breakdown was in the medical files. It was a significant moment in my health and I needed to talk. He was brilliant. I told him I had had suicidal thoughts, but I knew I would not act on them, given my long history with mental health and having never actively taken that option. I had a plan in place, with therapy and meditation, I wanted to rest and did not want chemical help, and he agreed that was a good plan of action but to check in with him the following week.

I had to nestle down and implement a complete gear change. And I finally got to speak to Samantha. I told her what had happened, and we discussed her coming down as soon as possible. I hadn't seen any of my family for nearly three years, and I needed to. I also told Ligita, and I cleared everything out of my diary and lay on my sofa for months, taking care of my boys and me and going with the flow. I ditched social media and hardly answered my phone. I told my work colleagues what had happened and that I couldn't do anything. I was going to tune in to me and see how I would best function, and I knew I needed to put the emergency brakes on.

In the stopping, I started to hear my intuition slowly, my spirit speaking to me, and I started the long journey back to myself. Firstly I started to read my angel cards daily. They were a gift from my friend, Phillippa, for my last birthday and are one of my favourite gifts ever because they keep giving and giving. They offer spiritual guidance and great tools for bringing positivity into your life. Whether you believe what you pick out is meant for you or not, be assured they are all meant for you. All you need to do is take the advice and implement the practices they teach.

This breakdown, I learned, was a massive breakthrough, a clear warning sign that I could not carry on as I had been. I had to allow myself to unmask and start tapping into my true autistic self, to start operating from my genuine authenticity, not one that I had created. I, a vulnerable, wounded, scarred individual who had suffered so much trauma at the hands of friends, boyfriends, relations, work and the media, had to strip it all back and take it one day at a time.

After the breakdown, my sense of self escaped me, slowly and without fanfare; I had no concept of how I looked, how I wanted to dress or who I was, and I even stopped exercising. My body was tired, and I just went with it.

Mum and Samantha came to see me. The boys went with Daniel so I could talk freely to my family. I was a complete mess when they arrived. I had been speaking to Mum on the phone over Christmas and New Year, the run-up to the breakdown, so when she arrived I was surprised when she asked me, 'What's been going on?' 'I've told you everything, Mum; it doesn't go away when I put the phone down.' Maybe it's out of sight, out of mind, or maybe it's because, historically, I looked like I always bounced back, and the belief being none of it had cost me anything emotionally.

And maybe that was my fault. Perhaps I hadn't explained myself adequately. I believed I had nobody to catch me, so I didn't ask for help. I had to steam ahead alone. Samantha had no idea of the pain I had suffered, so it was good to let it all out and have support from her. My beautiful big sister was back in my life and taking care of me, and it felt amazing.

When she left, she put a plan in place to check in with me every day, and I would tell her on a scale of nought to ten how I was feeling – nought being awful and ten being great. It was fantastic, and I felt someone was looking out for me from the family for the first time in years.

I was slowly getting better and making life changes in small increments. I was practising my meditation more frequently and starting to understand what had happened. I was doing okay, but what I wasn't doing was leaving the house. I went out only ever to buy food and get Valentino out to the charity shops or for a little walk – more for him than me.

My money was dwindling fast. Any money that came in was going on legal fees, rent and food, and I had to move home. I couldn't afford to stay, and I couldn't afford to go. My rent was exorbitant, and I couldn't do it any more. So I called Adam and told him my troubles. I was in the pits of my depression and could not see a way out. He said he would help me and put some money into my account.

With his help, I was able to reboot my life and start looking for a place. It was challenging to get out of the house and go and view properties, but I had to do it. I still lacked confidence, and when I looked in the mirror I couldn't see myself. I was a shell of me. I had no concept of how I looked or wanted to dress. I wore what I felt comfortable in, and that was leggings and sweatshirts that I kept finding in charity shops. It had somehow become my uniform. I needed comfort.

I got busy looking for a new place, and many people wanted to look at mine, so I started packing very early. I did not want strangers walking around my home knowing it was mine, so I hid anything personal and was surrounded by boxes for weeks, but it didn't bother me; in my heart, I had already left. I was clearing out everything I did not want or need any more and getting rid of the clutter, helping to clear my mind. Across all my moves, I had become highly skilled at getting rid of the stuff that no longer served me. It was a cleansing of sorts and had always helped me mentally in the past.

Whenever there was a viewing at the flat, I had to leave. I realised how agoraphobic I had become, so I would walk around the block and sit on the bench on the high street with the ever-present nagging feeling that someone might be taking a photograph of me right now, which was unnerving. I waited to get the call that I could return home out of the cold and back to safety.

Even viewing properties was stressful, all the shit you get told and the meeting strangers who had to take you around. I didn't need convincing and hated being 'sold' something. I didn't need help; I was letting my instincts be my guide. I know what I am looking for. I have always been like that in shops when buying clothes. I know what works for me, I don't need help and I'll ask for it if I do. I have always found it intrusive. I am opposed to their sales pitch. I like to gauge things for myself. I know people who don't see a movie or even read a book because some critic they don't know says they don't like it, thus cutting themselves off from an experience that they could have very well enjoyed.

After weeks of looking, I found a house. It felt right and safe and it was a great relief. I was getting out of central London for the first time in years. We needed a garden so that we could to step out and breathe, and I wanted to be closer to the children's paternal side of the family. The flat had been great all these years, but it was too small; we had all outgrown it, and I swore this would be my last rental ever. I had to sort my life out and put down some proper roots for the children and me.

During the search for a new home, my ADHD assessment also returned positive. I now had the full house. I was excited; finally I had the exact same diagnosis of my son, who had received his sixteen years before me. I could now get on with my life and get my head around what it means to juggle these conditions, and in the process understand as son better. Valentino was seventeen when I got my diagnosis. After all the years of caring for him, I now could really process what it meant to be autistic, and when I shared my news with him he simply said, 'Oh, that's interesting,' and it has been. Over the last year of my diagnosis we are closer than we have ever been, and what I see in him I now can see in me, having similar sensitivities, which is truly wonderful.

While convalescing, I talked to my spiritual friends and explored ideas about faith and wellness. One friend suggested I speak to a healer and psychic out in South Africa, and he offered to pay for the session for me as a gift, which I was learning was okay to accept and to do so graciously through my angel cards.

I arranged a Zoom with her, and she was brilliant and talked to me about my life and desires, and art kept coming up for her. She told me to read a book called *The Artist's Way* by Julia Cameron. It was another message of healing to embrace. I am a huge art lover and have been attracted to creative people my whole life and am interested in their process, and it was finally dawning on me why. It was because I, too, am creative in that way; I am an artist. I just had not tuned into that fully.

Julia Cameron advocates writing pages daily, in a stream of consciousness first thing in the morning, to get all your thoughts and feelings out of your head and on paper, and as a seasoned diarist this commitment felt good. I have not missed a day since, because this practice works. The work in her book is about tapping into your creative side, understanding why you are as you are and who you are, and unleashing what is dormant within. After the writing came the drawing, and it felt good.

The move date was 18 March, so before the big day I wanted to visit my family up North, see my dad, who I had missed, and reconnect with my Auntie Sue and Uncle Neil, whom I hadn't seen for many years. The journey might well have been to the top of Everest, such was the enormity of the mission. I had not been beyond my local high street for months, but I wanted to push myself and see what challenges the trip might hold. I was frightened to get a cab to the station, let alone be at the station and then get onto the train. I kept thinking one step at a time; I was like a small child; I had no guard, I just had a raw, vulnerable me. I was lucky that the train was not busy and so I had a decent experience. I just wrote, read and enjoyed the journey as I watched the ever-changing view pass by.

It was incredible to see my dad again, and I gave him the biggest hug I have ever given him. It was lovely to be home. Mum made delicious food and we watched telly and talked politics. I got to see most of the family. Sadly my aunt and uncle had Covid, so that visit was postponed.

The journey home was a shock to the system. The last train to London had been cancelled, so everyone who was meant to be on the previous one piled onto this one. It was bursting at the seams, and it got worse every time we made a stop. People were standing in the aisles everywhere; they were getting snappy and impatient with each other, and I could feel every niggle. I started experiencing shallow breaths.

Over the tannoy, the train guard asked if there was a doctor onboard as someone was ill, and we would stop at the next station to wait for an ambulance. The train was now filled to the rafters. I started contemplating whether I should try to get off and brave it. It took a while to psych myself up to get up, get my things and get out of there without drawing attention to myself. It would take a lot of courage, but if I'd stayed I knew I would have had a panic attack; it was rising, and I knew the ambulance would have to be used for me too. We sat at the station for about fifteen minutes, but I needed air and did not want the entire carriage looking at me while I did it. I was trying to keep myself small, minimise damage and get off the train without anybody noticing me. As soon I stood up to offer my seat to someone, she asked me loudly if I was Melanie Sykes. I whispered, 'Please don't shout it,' and I explained that I was struggling and did not want any attention drawn to me. Her mate told her to leave me alone, which I was grateful for, and she backed off.

I squeezed my way onto the platform, took a lungful of air, and set about finding another train to London. I realised I had done too much too soon and vowed I would not travel again for many months.

I spoke to my therapist about what happened and she suggested I put together an emergency kit with things that would help me in similar situations. So I started to pack a paper bag to breathe into, the best tool for a panic attack, which the nurse had shown me all those years ago, some written exercises for grounding, my CBD oil, prayer beads, a fan and aromatherapy oil to calm me when I went out. This little bag of tricks was my safety net, and even now I do not leave home without it.

What was apparent was that the agoraphobia was based on being out of practice with travelling due to the pandemic but also because I had started to unmask. I was no longer implementing all my bravery and bravado. My armour was melting away, and it was all excellent information, not because I did not want to get back to who I had been before the breakdown but so that I could accept who I was – an extremely sensitive person – and know that there was nothing wrong with that.

I had been ready for weeks, then finally the day of the move arrived. It was a beautiful sunny day, and I felt liberated. Adam, Ligita, me and all the removal men steamed into the day. During the move, Ligita and I lifted a laundry bag – she had one handle, and I had the other and, using my left arm, we swung it up and over to put it onto another bag. At that moment I suddenly felt a pop in my bicep. It was a peculiar sensation; it wasn't painful, but it hadn't felt right. I've got a high pain threshold anyway, so I just let it go and carried on with the move, lifting and carrying all day.

The new house was perfect for us, except there was no phone, Wi-Fi, doorbell or telephone line. It didn't even have basic TV channels. So I slowly brought the property back to life; it was challenging, but it had to be done. Adam came over and put up all my pictures and mirrors, and the following week was more unpacking and lifting, carrying and getting it right. Ligita and I worked hard to make it habitable. I needed to get it straight so I could continue to get well, and after a week of hard graft the house looked like I had lived there for years.

The weather was glorious, and I decided to lie in the garden and feel the sun's heat on my body; while relaxing, I realised that my left arm was not right; it hurt like hell.

'I think I should go to A&E,' I said to Ligita.

I waited hours for an x-ray. There was no break; I explained I had felt it in my bicep, but the pain was manifesting all around the elbow, and I could no longer make a pincer shape with my thumb and forefinger. Finally, the nurse said I might have torn a tendon and suggested I probably had severe tennis elbow. He put me in a sling and said maybe get a scan on it in a week or two if it doesn't feel better.

It did not get better, and I was not resting it as much as I should. I finally saw an osteopath, who stuck an acupuncture needle right into the elbow. I screamed the surgery down and thought I would hit the ceiling. He strapped me up and told me to rest. The problem was it was Easter, and Roman was home from university, so I was looking after both boys and doing too much.

It was just another sign from the universe that I had to slow down further, but it felt impossible. I went down to make dinner for us all and opened the cupboard to get a heavy pan out, and I couldn't do it. I looked at it and started to cry. First I was mentally screwed, and now I was physically screwed. How was I going to do this? I struggled to get dressed, wash my hair or get around the house. I was waiting for a miracle and feeling like I couldn't take any more. I could barely sleep, it hurt so much, and in the morning my arm would be completely numb and I couldn't move it; I wasn't taking care of it, and I needed some drastic action to get me through this.

I couldn't do everything I was supposed to, all the emails and fielding calls. However, I felt mentally strong enough to dabble in specific projects, and my new agent was doing what was needed. I also wanted to write this book and needed to write a proposal to show publishers, but I could not type one-handed. I also needed to apply for benefits to help keep me afloat, and dealing with forms online was another difficulty. It all felt impossible.

The big lesson emerging was gratitude. I was happy it wasn't my right arm, as that would have been a million times worse, and I had a whole new respect for my body. A moment of feeling not able-bodied is a wake-up call and a reminder that these things – my body – need to be respected.

I felt ready to get some ideas off the ground and pick up from where I'd left off work-wise. My desire for a podcast was strong, and I wanted to start working on my documentary ideas again and keep my magazine alive. So I talked to my agent, and he began to put the feelers out.

I agreed to appear on a few podcasts here and there and, if I said yes, to go on Tony Pitts and John Bishop's podcast, *Three*

Little Words. I chose autism, sex and death for my words. They could have been any words at this point; I wanted to share my ideas about everything. I sat there, my arm freshly in a sling, and waxed lyrical about my chosen topics, and I enjoyed the freedom. I no longer cared how my words would be twisted. I finally realised that I was in control of my narrative. As long as people could be bothered to return to the source, they would now hear it straight from the horse's mouth. I spoke of my breakdown publicly for the first time, but I believe it was edited out.

I was still exploring doing a podcast of my own, and when the opportunity arose I was interested. Things seemed to be working, and I was finally getting to where I had worked hard to get to, and I was excited about the future.

Chapter 22

I was drowning in admin and domestic commitments, and I could not get to my creative endeavours or even find space to think. Moreover, my arm had got worse and had put me on my arse, and I had to work things out, not wallow, but find solutions to get back up.

My angel cards had been coming up with similar messages about asking for help, something I rarely did. I'd read and realised that hyper independence was a trauma response, and I started to understand what that meant. Mainly because whenever I had trusted anybody to help me in the past, they had more often than not shafted me. It was a startling realisation that my uber independence was not all it was cracked up to be. In financial terms it was a good thing, but emotional independence it was not. I had convinced myself it was something to be proud of, but I realised it was a defence mechanism to protect me from hurt and further disappointment. So I needed to shift in my pattern, act on the direction received, and reach out to someone who could help me.

I asked a friend if she knew someone who would make a good PA. When she said yes, I was delighted. Historically I had limiting beliefs around having help personally. It felt like a 'grand' thing to have, but now it was a necessity. I needed someone to do the paperwork and organise my admin while I got on with my creative endeavours.

My PA was a wonderful, warm, funny Yorkshire woman who helped me so much, made me laugh, and took all my painful chores so I could get on with work. Now I just needed a hand around the house, and Ligita suggested a friend who lived locally who might be available to help me manage the home, cook, and be my left arm, domestically speaking, while I got stronger.

Over the next weeks this team of women carried some of the burden of my difficulties so I could continue to heal and branch out. I was starting to understand how blessed I was and focused on how I had been helped throughout my life. I was experiencing gratitude, and it wasn't something I needed to learn; it was just happening.

One Sunday, I was in a taxi with the boys on the way back from their grandparents when the driver helped me to see even more light. He asked what I had done to my arm, and when I told him the story, he said, 'Are you feeding it to help it heal?' It was an excellent question that I hadn't even considered. I'd been eating crap for months and hadn't even thought about fuelling my injury with the nutrition it needed to repair. Of course, I knew what I ate was essential to my health, but I was flabbergasted at myself for not even thinking of it.

I was so grateful to him, and as soon as I got home I rang my nutritionist friend Rhiannon Lambert and told her everything.

She knew I didn't have any money, so she set me up with an assessment as a gift, the beautiful angel that she is, and I accepted. I got all my 'bloods' done through my GP to see if I was deficient in anything, but thankfully they came back all well, except I needed to incorporate some extra calcium into my diet.

We chatted about my recent medical history and the breakdown, and I asked him why he wasn't pushing me to take HRT like every doctor had done at times before. I asked him purely out of curiosity, and he said that whatever I was doing was working, so why did I need it? He went on to say that it is a natural transition that has always been there, but our lifestyles have become so unnatural that we don't seem to be able to cope with it.

So many factors of your health come into play around menopause, but your lifestyle is key. You can't whitewash a number of conditions with one title. Some may not belong to it. You must break down the issues, what you can cope with and what you need help with to change. For example, I was waking up with anxiety on my chest, which I was told was a menopause symptom, so I knew not to say yes to it. I didn't have to buy into it, because it wasn't real, I could breathe it out. I also had hot flushes, which I learned to handle by using a fan, adjusting my bedding, wearing suitable breathable fabrics and always wearing layers. If I needed to strip down or pull on clothes, I could. I don't need HRT to tackle that; I just need to practise common sense.

Unfortunately, the 'symptoms' of menopause have been made into an industry that works from fearmongering. There is awareness, and then there is blanket brainwashing, and for the love of and pursuit of sanity we must find a middle ground.

I still was not venturing out, except sometimes if I had someone with me, so when I found myself with a free weekend, as Valentino had gone to Daniel's, I decided to take my SOS kit, brave the Tube, get myself into central London and go and see some art. The next morning I got up and got ready, feeling excited I was going out, but when I finally got to the front door I could not step through it. I literally could not get out of the door. I completely froze and then started to panic. This fed right into my claustrophobia, and my shallow breathing kicked in, so I called a friend I trusted to vent it all out. And in doing so I calmed down. Still, I was devastated. Who am I? Where had the old me gone? That person who had only ever been out there alone. It seemed I wasn't going anywhere fast, so I got back into my comfy clothes, got back onto my sofa and assured myself this was not forever; it was just for now. I had just tried too soon.

My injury was feeling pretty grizzly, and the pain was terrible at night, so I used a CBD cream and tried to keep on top of the pain instead of taking addictive painkillers that made me sick in other ways. My home was the centre of my universe. It was a rehab centre, my workplace, my study place and the focus of my family life. So I was reading exciting literature about all human conditions, about inflammations being signs of emotional distress and lots about trauma. I was picking up some interesting books in my local charity shops and reading some of Deepak Chopra's spiritual teachings and Jay Shetty's *Think Like a Monk*, which were inspiring. I was lost in novels, too, keeping fiction as always for escapism and educating myself on all the things that interest me, and reading books where the authors had an exquisite ability to express the beauty of the natural world in words.

I could escape to these incredible landscapes from the confines of my home and relish the sentence forms and the musicality within them. It was great for my soul; I was taking time and rebuilding.

My study dictated my feelings, and I was grateful for the pause. The universe was definitely taking care of that. I was starting to say yes to appearing on more podcasts and realising that communication is one of my skills, so I loved the medium.

My autistic nature was also coming to the fore, and I realised just how sensitive I was, for example to layers of sound, and how easily distracted I could be by movement in my eye line. I didn't like Zoom calls with more than two people; all the faces were a distraction, and I felt like I was being watched and struggled to juggle the conversation. So I started to ask for what I needed.

Women that ask for certain boundaries can be misconstrued as difficult. Many men ask for what they want, which is great, but we should be allowed the same courtesy. It is our right to equality. But if you challenge their status quo, you are considered a problem. It's ridiculous, and it's something I'm determined to see change. Men do not talk to other men the way they speak to women because they would be in deep danger of getting punched on the nose if they did.

Not all men, but quite a few, save up all their anger and anxiety and unleash it on women. Wherever we go, there is a permanent misogynistic structure in every setting. Even my late diagnosis and women's late diagnosis in general shines a light on girls' enforced conformity from an early age to do what is expected of them and their keen ability to mask any 'unwanted' behaviours. Boys can let it out and be who they are, resulting in their behavioural freedom, which reveals diagnoses earlier. This injustice is wrapped around some antiquated notion of 'boys will be boys'. These negative sexist beliefs leave millions of people unseen and, ultimately, generations of wounded people in their wake. And it's not just late diagnosis that is an issue – misdiagnosis can be equally, if not more, destructive for someone. For too long, women who don't fit a notion of normal have been deemed 'mad' or 'crazy'.

That said, a considerable female energy shift is happening, which sadly results in increased domestic abuse numbers, but this is a direct reaction to women knowing their worth. This is good news, and we must not stop the charge.

We are the only ones who can make that happen. We must keep asking for what we need and continue to establish boundaries. We can all operate better when we're in the right environment, and there's no reason why things cannot change at work and home.

I talked to my friends, colleagues and other women I have met about how men speak to them, and how they have been disrespectfully treated. The responses were all versions of the stories that have been shared here. I could write a book about the subtle everyday ways the patriarchy has affected me: mansplaining, undermining and derogatory comments have tainted everyday life. I once had a beautiful, tall, blonde bank manager at my local branch who told me that she was struggling to get higher in rank because she would be seen as a 'distraction' at work. This is not Victorian Britain; this is happening now. And because these big babies with uncontrollable drives lose their ability to think when a good-looking woman is around, they are given positions of power. When in fact they are powerless. Why aren't they being investigated and helped? We should not be flattened by men's inability to control themselves.

I still get inflamed by this, but anger is not the way. Open conversations must be had, and women need to speak up. But we must meet it with patience. Men have years of indoctrination into this mindset. It seems that men are completely lost now; they know that we are on the rise and they are not finding it easy. It's not because we want to be better or above anyone, but it's because we want equality. I know I do. That's all I've ever wanted, not to live under the cosh of the patriarchy but to rise up and become equals and friends.

Some people expect me to be the same person they thought I was before my public diagnosis. But these new 'labels' were huge for me. I learned about all the masks I had been using, and I was letting them drop. I was saying what I needed and could only broadcast on my terms, but I wasn't being heard. Production companies would say the same old spiel, and I was supposed to lap it up. I have seen that industry from every angle possible, so there is hardly anything I don't already know or haven't already seen. It felt like, 'Yeah, we know all that, but you are the same Melanie Sykes, I was now her with labels, but the rules were the same.

I have watched people trying to manipulate me into doing things I did not want to do, and they seemed to think I couldn't see it or feel it. It was extraordinary. I asked for what I needed, but no one was listening. It was fascinating to dip my toe back into the entertainment industry waters after some time out following my diagnosis, but still, the temperature was the same as it had always been, with no sensitivity around autisic me and my needs, even though now they all knew about it.

Everyone cared about what they could get out of it only; it was shocking.

I pulled the plug on the podcast and on having contractual relationships with these people and these projects and decided to pursue my future work differently, to break down the existing systems and find a way to spread my good messages.

Spurred on by the teachings of *The Artist's Way*, I enrolled on a watercolour class at a local tennis club. I smiled when the cabbie dropped me outside as I struggled to get out with one arm in a sling. He probably wondered, how the hell can she play tennis?

The art room overlooked the courts, and the sound of the tennis balls was soothing. I listened and watched the teacher, then set up, ready to start. In the first class we learned how to paint the sky. The teacher was helpful, and the other artists were lovely and I learned a lot. I borrowed a tearsheet from the teacher of a beach scene with a mother and child dancing on the shoreline at sunset and decided to try to paint it. I borrowed a few brushes, as the ones I had were not quite right, and I went for it. I love the colours, the energy, but mostly what it means.

When I got home I was so happy. I cried tears of gratitude and happiness. The lesson had given me a new set of eyes. I looked up at the sky, and in what I used to perceive as a grey sky I now saw pinks and purples. The atmosphere became so magical, with so many colours to observe. I was grateful for my new view and proud that I had braved something new and got out there. That first painting I did is still my favourite painting, and even though it was not finished I framed it, and it hangs by my bed and never fails to make me smile.

The painting class was the only thing that got me out over the next few weeks, and I was enjoying the therapy, the expression and the learning. However, I had had a distinct lack of exercise since January, and since the breakdown I hadn't put a foot inside a gym, I hadn't done any training or yoga at all, I was building a bit of a Buddha belly, and I didn't have much energy.

I was also mourning the loss of my body – but this was all just a process. Of course, my mental health had to come first, but it was wrapped up in my yoga and with my training. It was weird to not have these adrenaline boosters in my life. I didn't want to lose it entirely, but my arm didn't feel like it belonged to me. It had been in the sling too long. I visited a local osteopath who told me it was a 'massive' injury and that I had torn my bicep and the tendons. I was under her care now, and she was brilliant.

The friends around me also started to encourage me to look around the nearest town shops. I agreed and got some bits for the house. I couldn't believe how fragile I felt with everyone. I had not been out like this for a long time. I needed help to carry things, people to sit with me when I needed a rest. It was like learning to walk again.

We started going for walks so I could reconnect with nature, and we talked about spiritual teachings and ideas. I began decluttering my paperwork and got rid of old letters and photographs from and of people who were no longer in my life. I was doing regular salt baths in candlelight and playing beautiful music around the house – piano, violin, brass bands and orchestras. All things that made me feel good and that I had been guided to do by my angel cards.

I was starting to understand my diagnosis more every day. I'm a quiet person, and then I can be really loud. I get very excited when talking about something I'm passionate about and become highly animated. I also occasionally say things that are deemed just a bit out there, and there are things I've blurted out to be provocative, especially when drunk. My autism and ADHD mean I crave peace but am hardwired to be productive and these two conflicting conditions jostle for my attention. Thankfully all the breathing and meditation practices help me massively.

One day I got a call from Riccardo, who I hadn't spoken to since his last visit over. He was getting on with his life and so was I, but we were still friends, and it was all cool. He asked me if I wanted a surprise, and I told him I hated them. 'Well, I'm in London. I'd love to see you this afternoon,' he said. I felt a little bit miffed and a bit shocked. I had a meeting at 11, so I asked him to come at 1pm. When he arrived, he stood there with a beautiful smile and a gorgeous bunch of flowers, and we hugged, caught up, laughed and talked; I cried, as I always do, and he made us lunch. He told me he had a few days off the next month, and I suggested it might be nice for us to go and do something. We agreed that we might go to Rome. I'd been challenged just going into London, let alone going to an airport and then a flight, but I thought I had to do it at some point. *I've got three weeks to prepare mentally, and he will be at the other end. I can do this.* We had a few hours together, and then Riccardo was gone. I still hate surprises, but I realised sometimes they can be wonderful.

I was booked on the daft early flight to Venice – Riccardo and I had decided against Rome, preferring to avoid a city break and go to the Dolomites instead. The whole process was daunting. I explained to the driver that I hadn't travelled for a while and was suffering from agoraphobia. He was lovely and told me he had a family member who had suffered the same condition for years, so he was very understanding. I did a meditation in the car and kept my breathing consistent.

The airport wasn't too bad but managing my luggage with one arm was pretty dreadful, but I did ask for help where necessary. Finally, I got on the plane and was in the window seat. I felt hemmed in and somewhat cramped, and I started to feel a panic attack rise before we even took off. I spoke to the stewardess and she brought me a bottle of water. I took a sip and started using my beads and mantra, and mercifully I fell asleep and woke up when we were airborne. The second hurdle cleared.

Riccardo picked me up at the airport. I was happy to get there and had to decompress as he drove for five hours weaving through the mountain pass. It was heavenly. I felt humble amongst the views and inspired by the greatly expanding vistas that rose up ahead and around the car. I had not experienced anything like this for a long time and felt energised.

For the next few days I tuned into the birds, drank in the air and devoured the visual feast. I painted, meditated and read, and we walked. I was proud of myself for getting this far. I had a few days in Venice before I returned home, giving me a top-up of its magic, which always filled my soul. My arm was on the home straight of recovery too, and my brilliant osteopath guided me back to the gym and physio; sadly, there was no chance of yoga as yet, but one step at a time. Finally, she released me from her care with the encouragement that I could go it alone.

Getting the ball rolling on my documentary was a priority. I was now in conversation with a director whose film I had seen through watching my BAFTA screeners.

I contacted him on social media to tell him I thought his work was brilliant, and he responded. I was thrilled that he took the time to acknowledge my message, and I believe it is always important to let people know how they impact you positively. Of course, you mustn't expect anything in return, but it is a delightful feeling if something does come back.

I still wanted to make the autism documentary and I finally felt well enough to start thinking about that again. It was time to start picking up these conversations. I got to speak more about making a film and told him what I'd experienced in the mainstream television world, how their view was blinkered and formulaic. It was about airtime, dumbing down, viewing figures and money, not about the subject matter itself and the activism that would be ignited if the programme was powerful enough. They didn't have the grand vision that I had. If I was going to make it, I had to make it independently. The director I was speaking to began to give me advice here and there, and I took it and kept running with his ideas, and he also told me that to get the film's final cut I had to direct it myself.

At first I thought, no way, how can I direct it? But as soon as I felt that, I pulled myself back and, in a second, flipped it to 'Yeah, why can't I? I can do anything I want.' He told me about a documentary film festival in Sheffield the following month and that I should get a ticket and we could go together. I was nervous and out of my comfort zone, but I had to challenge myself for the greater good. So I bought my tickets, met him in a car park in North London one Sunday morning, and we headed to Sheffield, having never met before.

We got on extremely well. I felt like I'd known him all my life. He's brilliant, tells a good yarn, and talks more than anybody I know. It was terrific. We did a bit of networking, which I found challenging, but he supported me, and we went to see some exciting talks, and I saw some interesting films and met some proactive people and made some important connections.

I have so many missions and things I want to achieve. I am creating new levels of opportunity for myself and letting my instincts guide me towards a future that makes me happy – and hopefully will help other people along the way too.

Outro

I'm still slowly stretching my boundaries since my diagnosis and seeing how they feel in all areas of my life. I will never be how I once was; I will never go back to the pace at which I was going and the trauma after trauma of communicating with people who did not see me. I've unmasked, and now I'm taking my time making decisions about what I agree to do, and ensuring my boundaries are at play in all areas of my life. I have unearthed how super sensitive I am and I am respecting it and feeling well.

I am also now on a private prescription for medical cannabis. I have the oil I ingest in the morning and again in the afternoon, and in the evenings, if I feel like it, I inhale the flower burned in a dab pen. Within one week these small, controlled amounts have calmed my nervous system and cleared my mind. Now that I have experienced its healing powers, I want to shatter old narratives about cannabis and spread the word about the good it can do, to open people's minds to what is rightfully ours. Natural medicine belongs to us.

I listen to my inner voice all the time now. Sometimes it's mine, and sometimes it's a line I have read or heard, a message that has resonated, and I act on that – Bruce Lee's 'Be like water' words were very useful to me, to name just one.

We must be open to change and never become stagnant. We can move into what we like when we listen to our hearts, souls and guts. Our inner voice talks to us all day, every day. It is your unique internal satnav and is there to guide you to safety.

As I have written this story, I can now see all the signs I ignored. How misguided I have been. I believe without all these detours I wouldn't have found the wisdom. These lessons have been unnerving to recollect, but I now know I needed them to know where I stand.

I enjoy a private life, and I've worked hard to have one. I will now only use my profile to help others. I, like everybody, need to earn a living and feather my nest, but my new work will have meaning. No more tap dancing for cooperations who couldn't give two hoots about my well-being. I'm going to live a centred and grounded life of service.

And despite all I have shared, if you've ever seen me smile on TV or heard me laugh on the radio, be assured I was not faking it. At that moment, that was how I felt. It was real. Mostly, though, my struggle behind the scenes of showbiz and media was burdensome on my heart, and dealing with the gargantuan egos of those in charge, mixed with some of the stars' attitudes and snottiness, was abhorrent and torturous for me.

I am my own power source; I do not need to find it in other people or places. I am more concerned with creating a life for myself. I have been wounded by the narrative in the press that has said that I am only interested in people for their money, youth, a 'toyboy', a plaything, or someone's status, which I never see anyway. I've been painted as somebody who uses people, and that injustice used to gall. But I am over it now, and I realise that it is them that have been using me.

If you like reading tabloid shite and weekly gossip magazines, stop and see how your life will change. These things are only there to make money for the cooperation and make you feel angry, weak, judgemental and easy to control. Photographers should not be allowed to stalk women and, worse, do it when they are with their children, but it will continue if the thirst for it prevails.

My eldest son stopped walking down the street with me from a young age, which obviously concerned me, but I could not blame him. What child wants to be photographed on the way to school? Even into his teenage years he would not go out to eat with me, scared of the intrusion it may bring. The impact of these tabloids is profound. It's not just a photo for your approval or bile; it's people's lives.

Step away, take a lungful of air and start looking within; look at your family, your community. What can you do to make the world a better place? We have so much power collectively. It's the only power we have. You are being lied to, and if they have the time and inclination to lie about little old me, then they are definitely lying about everything else.

I've been growing as a person, appreciating myself properly for the first time in my life, all while I've been writing this book. I now feel I can start to celebrate myself, which is something that has always eluded me until now. We should always celebrate even the smallest achievements and mine for our endless potential.

We all can be reborn, but first we need to take care of ourselves; look after the child inside of us. Not poison ourselves with a toxic history, but set ourselves free from their bonds, reform and re-emerge. Think freely, be spirited and go with your intuition. Turn off that phone, turn off your TV and connect with yourselves. Go for a walk, say hello to your dark side, look at the regrets and hurts, and break and rebuild. If you don't break it open before you die, you're not really living.

My sobriety definitely kickstarted my awareness and journey onto my current and future path. Finally, I could see things clearly, which was powerful but by no means easy. I was peeling away the layers of ego and stories of defence, breaking them open. I got to see people more clearly, but mostly I had clarity about myself. I love, I've always loved, but I have given chunks of myself away to people and neglected myself. Getting sober was my first act of self-love: no more hiding and making excuses. I pulled myself up by my bootstraps and yanked myself away from all my shit and shame. My self-worth has finally been revealed to me at the age of fifty-two, and I will not let that go.

Who are you hiding from? Yourself? What good is that? We must live for today with all its magic. We must be spontaneous, not regimented. Go with the flow of our spirit. You have heard the old saying that this is not a dress rehearsal, well, from my experience in showbiz, dress rehearsals are never as good as the real thing. The spontaneity is where the magic happens, and it is the same in life. You have to crack yourself open. Look at all the nooks and crannies, and face the hurt and shame that will be there. It is the only way to truly live. We are all equal and we all belong to this world in equal measure. Do not let anybody tell you any different.

I am learning new things about myself every day, acting on whatever feels good and walking away from what doesn't, without looking back with anger, hurt and guilt.

I care about Daniel, the father of my children, and I always will, and despite everything we have produced the most incredible children.

I am grateful for those who have passed, my beautiful family and friends; their words of wisdom and love reside within me in their deaths. I speak to them and feel their presence every day. Their good messages live within me always.

My diagnosis was the last of the big revelations about myself, the missing pieces of my life, the access to the map to find myself.

Although unique and beautiful, the journey since has been rough; I've had nowhere to hide. I had to do the work to understand myself fully. I had to graft and graft hard. It has taken a lot of energy to go back and to remember, to realise and forgive myself for everything. Everything I've thought, done or said — and mostly, what I've done to myself.

I believe efficiency around people getting diagnosis should change, and the narrative around it should be more mainstream. Everything you hear is from a neurotypical perspective, and the clinician's spiel around autism is also based on decades-old theories that need to be abolished. Early diagnosis is crucial, and the neurotypical world needs to bend to accommodate it all. We must be more inclusive; stop telling us it's your way or the highway and stop telling us how we are without asking or letting us be the front, middle and centre of the narrative.

I could sit here wondering if only I had known about my autism and ADHD when I was little, what might have been different. Understanding some of my behaviour, my overachieve mode, my capacity to tell the truth, my obvious seeking of solace in drink to numb my sensitivities – which I now know are my strengths. And how alcohol impaired my vision and disabled my internal barometer, robbing me of my ability to gauge the temperature of what was good for me. I have suffered abuse, blackmail, addiction, and all the fallout from these, but I understand I needed to go down every one of those roads. That was and is my destiny. I needed to learn everything to help others – to encourage diagnosis and to break down the systems that currently surround it.

I still have many years left on this road, and from now on I will walk it with authenticity – no more pretending, no more hiding. I will move forward. I will be my guide, I will be my own warm, loving embrace, use the force of my ever-growing faith, and extend it to all things and beings. In learning gratitude I have unearthed my need to master patience, and it is through truths revealed that I come to this.

I hope my words have inspired you to make the changes you need to evolve your life and live every second in the light of its blessing.

Much love
Melanie.

Acknowledgements

Thank you to my agent, Cathryn Summerhayes, backing my desire to write this book myself.

To my editor, Genevieve, for understanding the delicacy that is writing a memoir and your support throughout.

Thank you Tony Pitts for the inspiration. You are one of my kind.

Jojo Moyes, you are my angel.

To Eileen Cooper, your work beams from my book, a beacon of hope and light. It has been so incredible to get to know you over these last few years.

To Lucy at Champneys, Tring, thank you for your energy whilst I wrote the first draft of this book. What a woman you are.

To Adam, more tears of laughter to come my friend. It's what we do. Thank you.

To all the creatives in the world that have lifted me in my many hours of need. I salute you.

And lastly my boys, I could not be prouder of you and my love and gratitude for you is eternal.

Harper
North

Book Credits

HarperNorth would like to thank the following staff and contributors for their involvement in making this book a reality:

Laura Amos

Hannah Avery

Fionnuala Barrett

Luke Bird

Samuel Birkett

Claire Boal

Caroline Bovey

Ciara Briggs

Katie Buckley

Sarah Burke

Alan Cracknell

Jonathan de Peyer

Anna Derkacz

Tom Dunstan

Kate Elton

Simon Gerratt

Monica Green

Graham Holmes

Ben Hurd

Megan Jones

Jean-Marie Kelly

Taslima Khatun

Nic & Lou

Ben McConnell

Alice Murphy-Pyle

Adam Murray

Genevieve Pegg

Agnes Rigou

James Ryan

Florence Shepherd

Zoe Shine

Emma Sullivan

Katrina Troy

Daisy Watt

Kelly Webster

Tom Whiting

For more unmissable reads,
sign up to the HarperNorth newsletter at
www.harpernorth.co.uk

or find us on Twitter at
@HarperNorthUK

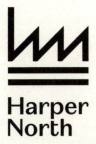

Harper
North

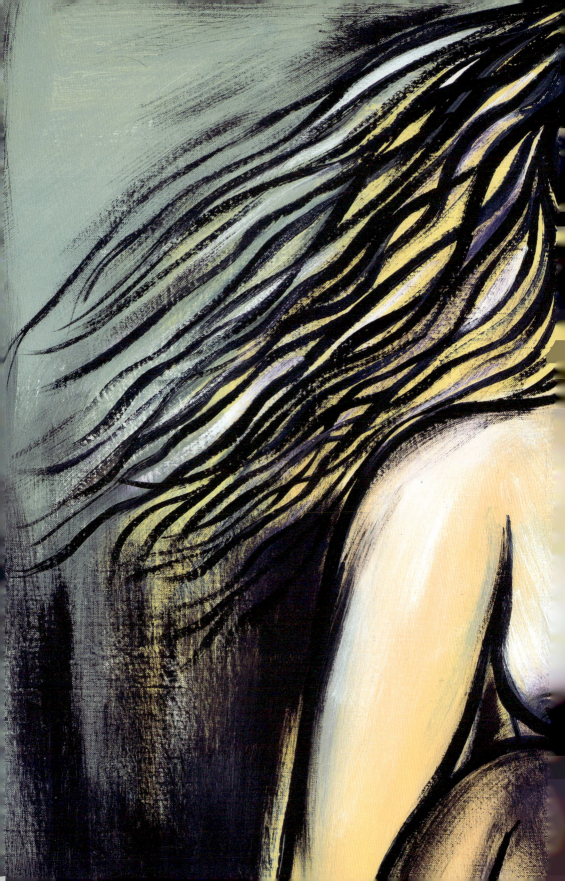